Becoming a Better Physician

Mark Allan Goldstein • Kathy May Tran
Editors

Becoming a Better Physician

Insightful and Inspirational Stories from Attending Physicians, Residents, and Medical Students

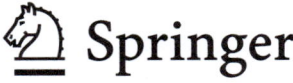

Editors
Mark Allan Goldstein
Adolescent and Young Adult Medicine
Department of Pediatrics
Massachusetts General Hospital
Boston, MA, USA

Kathy May Tran
General Internal Medicine
Department of Medicine
Massachusetts General Hospital
Boston, MA, USA

Department of Pediatrics
Harvard Medical School
Boston, MA, USA

Department of Medicine
Harvard Medical School
Boston, MA, USA

ISBN 978-3-031-69412-7   ISBN 978-3-031-69413-4   (eBook)
https://doi.org/10.1007/978-3-031-69413-4

© The Editor(s) (if applicable) and The Author(s), under exclusive license to Springer Nature Switzerland AG 2024
This work is subject to copyright. All rights are solely and exclusively licensed by the Publisher, whether the whole or part of the material is concerned, specifically the rights of translation, reprinting, reuse of illustrations, recitation, broadcasting, reproduction on microfilms or in any other physical way, and transmission or information storage and retrieval, electronic adaptation, computer software, or by similar or dissimilar methodology now known or hereafter developed.
The use of general descriptive names, registered names, trademarks, service marks, etc. in this publication does not imply, even in the absence of a specific statement, that such names are exempt from the relevant protective laws and regulations and therefore free for general use.
The publisher, the authors and the editors are safe to assume that the advice and information in this book are believed to be true and accurate at the date of publication. Neither the publisher nor the authors or the editors give a warranty, expressed or implied, with respect to the material contained herein or for any errors or omissions that may have been made. The publisher remains neutral with regard to jurisdictional claims in published maps and institutional affiliations.

This Springer imprint is published by the registered company Springer Nature Switzerland AG
The registered company address is: Gewerbestrasse 11, 6330 Cham, Switzerland

If disposing of this product, please recycle the paper.

"Often after I have gone into my office harassed by personal perplexities of whatever sort, fatigued physically and mentally, after two hours of intense application to the work [writing], I came out at the finish completely rested (and I mean rested) ready to smile and to laugh as if the day were just starting. That is why as a writer I have never felt that medicine interfered with me but rather that it was my very food and drink, the very thing which made it possible for me to write."

William Carlos Williams M.D.,
pediatrician and general practitioner,
writer and poet 1883–1963
The Practice in *The Doctor Stories*

Foreword

In the spring of 2020, I was practicing primary care internal medicine and serving as a mentor for healthcare workers interested in writing. When the COVID-19 pandemic began, I assumed that the demand for my mentorship would disappear. Who among my colleagues would have the time or desire to write during a global health crisis? Surely setting thoughts on paper or computer screen was a luxury for which those busy trying to save lives would have little use.

How wrong I was.

By mid-March of that terrible year, more manuscripts and queries appeared in my inbox each week than I'd received in months. Hospital staff sent me essays, editorials, poems, and fragments of memoirs and novels. Some asked for writing prompts, questions that might inspire them to document their experiences of this extraordinary period, perhaps for publication, for their children and grandchildren to read one day, or simply for themselves. Many who emailed me drafts were doctors working on the front lines of the battle against the coronavirus in ICUs, emergency rooms, and makeshift COVID units. Several residents attended a weekly virtual writing workshop I organized shortly after the start of the pandemic. Some signed in while on duty at the hospital, scrawling or tapping out their stories while covered head to toe in protective gear.

These residents were joining a long and rich tradition. Hippocrates, Hildegard of Bingen, Anton Chekhov, William Carlos Williams, and Oliver Sacks are but a few of the physicians who have crafted narratives even—especially—in times of extreme difficulty and uncertainty including amid wars and plagues. Today, when the electronic medical record and increasing administrative duties make the practice of medicine feel more rushed and less reflective than in the past, and when caregiver burnout, medical disinformation, racial and gender inequity, environmental disaster, and political discord all loom like dark clouds over the exam room and hospital bedside, more physicians than ever are writing.

Combining doctoring with writing makes sense. Doctors have unique and intimate access to people's stories, and we understand deeply the power of storytelling to heal, educate, and expose injustice. Still, juggling the two activities has never been easy. Practicing medicine and writing each require much time and energy, though not in the same ways. The doctor moves briskly from stretcher to clinic to OR solving problems, while the writer works at a more contemplative pace. Doctors tend to be efficient, exacting, prone to perfectionism. Writers, in contrast, are creative, expansive, and tend to daydream. Indeed, doctoring and writing might be seen as such different pursuits as to be mutually exclusive. Chekhov's publisher thought so. In 1894, he urged the then young physician-writer to quit medicine altogether and write full-time, so as not to, as he put it, "chase after two hares at once." In the 1920s, Ezra Pound, using much the same logic, advised Williams to abandon his medical practice in Rutherford, New Jersey, live among the literati in Paris, and devote himself wholly to poetry.

Luckily for patients, and for readers, many physicians, including those whose essays appear in this volume, have chosen to "chase after two hares"—to practice medicine and also to write. These physician-writers seem to have concluded that the two activities aren't really in opposition to each another or even separable. Williams, who eschewed Pound's advice and continued doctoring and writing in New Jersey for decades, surely felt this way. When asked once how he sustained his passion for both medicine and writing he replied, "They amount for me to nearly the same thing."

The authors of the essays in this collection express the satisfactions and joys of medical practice while also exploring self-doubt, mental health challenges, ethical quandaries, and work–family balance and imbalance. In doing so they reveal personal vulnerabilities and quirks about which physician-writers of previous generations often remained silent.

The contributing authors work all over the United States, practice a variety of specialties, and are at different stages of their careers, from training to retirement. They are diverse storytellers telling diverse stories. What unites them is the conviction that storytelling, and writing in particular, can make a physician both more effective and more fulfilled. A chief concern of patients today is that doctors are too time-constrained and distracted by various tasks to listen to them. A chief concern among physicians today is that those same time constraints and distractions have lessened physicians' autonomy. Writing, as is evident in these pages, addresses both concerns, attuning physicians more keenly to patients' voices and also to our own.

This book offers no easy prescriptions to cure burnout or fix health care systems. The stories it contains will, however, move us, validate our experiences, and inspire us to find our own ways to improve the practice of medicine for patients and caregivers alike. I am deeply grateful to the physician-writers whose essays appear here. They have approached their work with intelligence, curiosity, honesty, and empathy—as the best writers and the best physicians always have.

Dr. Koven practiced primary care internal medicine for over 30 years at Massachusetts General Hospital and now serves as the hospital's Writer-in-Residence. She also co-directs the Media and Medicine program at Harvard Medical School. Her essay collection, *Letter to a Young Female Physician*, was published by W.W. Norton & Co. in 2021.

Writer-in-Residence, Massachusetts General Hospital   Suzanne Koven
Boston, MA, USA
Department of Medicine, Harvard Medical School
Boston, MA, USA
Department of Global Health and Social Medicine
Harvard Medical School, Boston, MA, USA

Preface

It seems that my best ideas come unsolicited and without warning. On a cool, damp, dreary spring morning in New England, I reviewed data in a report from the Massachusetts Medical Society regarding burnout among resident physicians. More than ¾ of the residents surveyed by the society reported symptoms of burnout. And 23% felt completely burned out and at a point that they would need to seek help.

Thinking back to my residency at Massachusetts General Hospital (MGH) decades ago, I recalled never having any symptoms that could have been burnout. So I had an idea for a book to help prevent burnout in trainees, contacted a senior editor at Springer, developed a proposal, and a book plan was approved.

The concept was to develop a book of essays for a medical audience at all stages of their careers, written by attending physicians, residents, and medical students. While burnout was the initial subject, the essay topics eventually were broadened to address personal and professional challenges the authors had experienced. These pieces would be personal reflections on the nature of the challenge, how the author responded to it, and how that response made them a better physician.

I needed help to accomplish this task. Coming with many accomplishments and numerous accolades, Dr. Kathy May Tran agreed to be co-editor. A medicine hospitalist at MGH, associate editor of the Case Records at the *New England Journal of Medicine,* and director of "Stories of the MGH," she was the perfect person to be the co-editor. Within a month, we had crafted an overall strategy, and then we commenced a whirlwind journey promoting our plans to peers, seeking contributors, and reviewing and revising essays.

This project has not only been a tremendous educational experience, but it has also provided us great joy. And we dearly hope that after reading these essays, the readership will gain insight, inspiration, and knowledge to confront the many challenges physicians face in their personal and professional lives.

Boston, MA, USA   Mark Allan Goldstein

Introduction

Medical school graduation is the beginning, not the end of a doctor's education. Over the course of a career, a physician never stops striving to learn more, to develop greater clinical judgment, to be *better*. But what does it mean to be a better physician? How do we become one?

One of the main ways physicians evolve is by dealing with obstacles. Long work days (and nights), difficult diagnostic dilemmas, and emotionally wrenching patient interactions routinely challenge the physician. But other, more personal hurdles can be even more formative.

This is a collection of essays by doctors and doctors-to-be, written for doctors and those interested in doctoring. Each describes an obstacle that the author faced, how they responded, and how the experience helped them become a better physician. Some stories are easy to celebrate, such as those about learning medicine, honing communication, forging relationships, and summoning the courage to speak up. Others, about living in poverty, navigating racism, battling addiction, getting fired, and facing death, are more painful to absorb. Each helped the storyteller grow in medicine and in life. We hope they will help the reader grow, too.

The authors of these essays are medical students, residents, fellows, attendings, and retired physicians. Some are bestselling authors, creators of award-winning storytelling series, and contributors to the *New England Journal of Medicine*, the *Journal of the American Medical Association*, *The New Yorker*, and *The New York Times*. Many, however, had not considered themselves storytellers before embarking upon this project. Among these are foundation presidents, hospital leaders, clinic directors, social media influencers, national and international activists, and the doctor next door. Through this project, all have realized their own stories.

As you read each themed chapter, opening commentary, and essay, we invite you to ponder the challenges that you have faced. How did you respond? What did you learn? How did it make you a better physician and a better person? What is your story?

Mark Allan Goldstein
Kathy May Tran

Contents

1 **Learning and Training** 1
  Mark Allan Goldstein, Bernard E. Trappey, Megan Marshall,
  Shan W. Liu, Trisha K. Paul, Victor A. Lopez-Carmen, and
  Minali Nigam
  Commentary: Thawing 2
  Good Grief 4
  The Night I Almost Walked Away from Medicine 6
  Work on Professionalism 8
  My Undeserved Coaches 11
  Married in Medicine 13

2 **Career** 17
  Kathy May Tran, Michael F. Bierer, Mai Uchida, Farrin A. Manian,
  Michelle L. Izmaylov, Erica C. Kaye, Joseph R. Betancourt,
  Andrea Reilly, and Michael Jellinek
  Commentary: My COVID Epitaph 18
  Finding Empathy While Fighting Misinformation 19
  No Silence, Please! 21
  Instead of That Phone Call 25
  Hard Work 27
  A Triumph Over Moral Injury 31
  Forging Trust 34
  Being Fired 37

3 **Caregiving** 41
  Kathy May Tran, Marc S. Weinberg, Susan Hata,
  Laya Jalilian-Khave, Michael Natter, Vinayak Venkataraman,
  Emmett A. Kistler, LaShyra T. Nolen, and Sandeep Jauhar
  Commentary: Deep Breath 42
  Befriending Our Edges 43
  The Art of Listening: Beyond Languages and Borders 45
  One to One 48
  Young Hearts Dying 50
  Tell Me More 54

Superheroes Need Healing Too.................................. 57
My Father Didn't Want to Live if He Had Dementia—But Then He
Had It 60

4 Physician as Patient 63
Mark Allan Goldstein, Paula K. Rauch, Carrie Cunningham,
Emily M. Herzberg, Rana L. A. Awdish, Emily Silverman,
Peter Grinspoon, Giuseppina Romano-Clarke, David V. Diamond,
and Evonne Kaplan-Liss
Commentary: There Is No "Us" and "Them" in the Doctor–Patient
Relationship 64
There Is No Crying in Surgery 65
I'll Never Float Again....................................... 68
The 7-Year Consult.. 70
Joy Machine 73
Free Refills 76
Doctors Are Humans: Breaking Painful Stereotypes 80
A Journey's Journal: Finding Strength in Words and Gratitude in
Experience.. 83
Lessons Learned 86

5 Personal Growth 91
Kathy May Tran, Michael Natter, Elizabeth Roux, Felippe
O. Marcondes, Cassie Craun Ferguson, Kamal R. Chémali,
Perry Pong, and Chi T. Viet
Commentary: Anatomy of Burnout 92
The Blessing of a Bear 92
unDOCumented Medicine 95
Overcoming Overwhelm...................................... 97
The Frustration of a Musician-Turned-Physician................... 100
Are you Chinese? Yes, and I'm Asian American Too 103
Embracing Loss to Find Fulfillment............................ 106

6 Love and Loss 109
Michael Jellinek, Kerri Palamara McGrath, Imani E. McElroy,
Mark Allan Goldstein, Maria Trent, Clara Baselga-Garriga,
and Gleeson Rebello
Commentary: Abe... 110
The Gifts Grief Brings: One Physician's Journey Through Grief
After Loss 110
Mental Compartment Syndrome: It Is Time to Decompress 113
No Symptoms or Signs....................................... 116
Learning to Live in an Alternate Universe 118
Superiority of the Grieving Syndrome (SGS)...................... 120
I Learned the Most from My Father's Death Following Surgery 123

Acknowledgements... 129

Index.. 131

Editors and Contributors

About the Editors

Mark Allan Goldstein, M.D. Dr. Goldstein practiced pediatrics, adolescent medicine, and family medicine for over 45 years in settings that included a rural health clinic adjacent to the Navajo reservation in New Mexico and academic medical centers in Boston, Massachusetts. He has taught countless medical students, residents, and fellows over his career. Dr. Goldstein's papers have appeared in the *New England Journal of Medicine*, *The Journal of Clinical Endocrinology & Metabolism*, the *Journal of Adolescent Health*, *Academic Psychiatry*, and other publications. He is the author, co-author, or editor of 18 books including *How Technology, Social Media, and Current Events Profoundly Affect Adolescents* (Oxford University Press).

Kathy May Tran, M.D. Dr. Tran is a Vietnamese American from the Deep South who serves patients and teaches trainees in the city of Boston, Massachusetts, and indigenous nations in Rosebud, South Dakota, and Kotzebue, Alaska. She prioritizes workforce well-being by leading programs for community building, music and medicine, diversity and equity, and storytelling—personal, professional, and academic. In addition to writing and editing the historic Case Records in the *New England Journal of Medicine*, Dr. Tran is the co-editor of *50 Studies Every Hospitalist Should Know* (Oxford University Press) and the founder and director of the storytelling series *Stories of the Massachusetts General Hospital*.

Contributors

Rana L. A. Awdish, M.D., M.S. Pulmonary Hypertension Program, Pulmonary and Critical Care, Department of Medicine, Henry Ford Health, Detroit, MI, USA

Department of Medicine, Michigan State College of Human Medicine, East Lansing, MI, USA

Department of Medicine, Wayne State University School of Medicine, Detroit, MI, USA

Clara Baselga-Garriga, M.F.A. Harvard Medical School, Boston, MA, USA

Joseph R. Betancourt, M.D., M.P.H. Commonwealth Fund, New York, NY, USA

General Internal Medicine, Department of Medicine, Massachusetts General Hospital, Boston, MA, USA

Department of Medicine, Harvard Medical School, Boston, MA, USA

Michael F. Bierer, M.D., M.P.H. General Internal Medicine, Department of Medicine, Massachusetts General Hospital, Boston, MA, USA

Department of Medicine, Harvard Medical School, Boston, MA, USA

Kamal R. Chémali, M.D. Department of Neurology, University Hospitals Cleveland Medical Center, Cleveland, OH, USA

Department of Neurology, Case Western Reserve University School of Medicine, Cleveland, OH, USA

Carrie Cunningham, M.D., M.P.H. Endocrine Surgery Program, Department of Surgery, Massachusetts General Hospital, Boston, MA, USA

Department of Surgery, Harvard Medical School, Boston, MA, USA

David V. Diamond, M.D. Medical Department, Massachusetts Institute of Technology, Cambridge, MA, USA

Cassie Craun Ferguson, M.D. Pediatric Emergency Medicine, Department of Pediatrics, Children's Wisconsin, Milwaukee, WI, USA

Department of Pediatrics, Medical College of Wisconsin, Milwaukee, WI, USA

Mark Allan Goldstein, M.D. Adolescent and Young Adult Medicine, Department of Pediatrics, Massachusetts General Hospital, Boston, MA, USA

Department of Pediatrics, Harvard Medical School, Boston, MA, USA

Peter Grinspoon, M.D. General Internal Medicine, Department of Medicine, Massachusetts General Hospital, Boston, MA, USA

Department of Medicine, Harvard Medical School, Boston, MA, USA

Susan Hata, M.D. Medicine-Pediatrics Residency Program, Massachusetts General Hospital, Boston, MA, USA

General Internal Medicine, Department of Medicine, Massachusetts General Hospital, Boston, MA, USA

Department of Pediatrics, Massachusetts General Hospital, Boston, MA, USA

Department of Pediatrics, Harvard Medical School, Boston, MA, USA

Emily M. Herzberg, M.D. Newborn Services, Department of Pediatrics, Massachusetts General Hospital, Boston, MA, USA

Department of Pediatrics, Harvard Medical School, Boston, MA, USA

Michelle L. Izmaylov, M.D. General Internal Medicine and Public Health, Department of Medicine, Vanderbilt University Medical Center, Nashville, TN, USA

Laya Jalilian-Khave, M.D. Department of Psychiatry, Yale School of Medicine, New Haven, CT, USA

Sandeep Jauhar, M.D., Ph.D. Cardiology, Department of Medicine, Northwell Health, New Hyde Park, NY, USA

Michael Jellinek, M.D. Child Psychiatry Service, Department of Psychiatry, Massachusetts General Hospital, Boston, MA, USA

Department of Pediatrics, Massachusetts General Hospital, Boston, MA, USA

Department of Psychiatry, Harvard Medical School, Boston, MA, USA

Evonne Kaplan-Liss, M.D., M.P.H. Center for Compassionate Communication, T. Denny Sanford Institute for Empathy and Compassion, University of California San Diego, San Diego, CA, USA

Department of Pediatrics, University of California San Diego Health, San Diego, CA, USA

Erica C. Kaye, M.D., M.P.H. Quality of Life and Palliative Care, Department of Oncology, St. Jude Children's Research Hospital, Memphis, TN, USA

Emmett A. Kistler, M.D., M.H.Q.S. Critical Care, Department of Medicine, Mount Auburn Hospital, Cambridge, MA, USA

Department of Medicine, Harvard Medical School, Boston, MA, USA

Suzanne Koven, M.D., M.F.A. Writer-in-Residence, Massachusetts General Hospital, Boston, MA, USA

Department of Medicine, Harvard Medical School, Boston, MA, USA

Department of Global Health and Social Medicine, Harvard Medical School, Boston, MA, USA

Shan W. Liu, M.D., S.D. Department of Emergency Medicine, Massachusetts General Hospital, Boston, MA, USA

Department of Emergency Medicine, Harvard Medical School, Boston, MA, USA

Victor A. Lopez-Carmen Medical School, Boston, MA, USA

Farrin A. Manian, M.D., M.P.H. Department of Medicine, Mercy Hospital-St. Louis, St. Louis, MO, USA

Department of Medicine, St. Louis University Medical School, St. Louis, MO, USA

Department of Medicine, Ponce Health Sciences University, St. Louis, MO, USA

Felippe O. Marcondes, M.D., M.P.H. General Internal Medicine, Department of Medicine, Massachusetts General Hospital, Boston, MA, USA

Department of Medicine, Harvard Medical School, Boston, MA, USA

Megan Marshall, M.D. Medicine-Pediatrics Residency Program, Massachusetts General Hospital, Boston, MA, USA

Imani E. McElroy, M.D., M.P.H. General Surgery Residency Program, Massachusetts General Hospital, Boston, MA, USA

Kerri Palamara McGrath, M.D. General Internal Medicine, Department of Medicine, Massachusetts General Hospital, Boston, MA, USA

Department of Medicine, Harvard Medical School, Boston, MA, USA

Michael Natter, M.D. Endocrinology, Diabetes, and Metabolism, Department of Medicine, New York University Langone Medical Center, New York, NY, USA

Department of Medicine, New York University Grossman School of Medicine, New York, NY, USA

Minali Nigam, M.D. Neurology Residency Program, Brigham and Women's Hospital, Boston, MA, USA

Neurology Residency Program, Massachusetts General Hospital, Boston, MA, USA

LaShyra T. Nolen, M.P.P. Harvard Medical School, Boston, MA, USA

Trisha K. Paul, M.D. Quality of Life and Palliative Care, Department of Oncology, St. Jude Children's Research Hospital, Memphis, TN, USA

Department of Hematology, St. Jude Children's Research Hospital, Memphis, TN, USA

Perry Pong, M.D. Education and Training, Charles B. Wang Community Health Center, New York, NY, USA

Department of Medicine, Weill Cornell Medical College, New York, NY, USA

Paula K. Rauch, M.D. Child Psychiatry Service, Department of Psychiatry, Massachusetts General Hospital, Boston, MA, USA

Department of Psychiatry, Harvard Medical School, Boston, MA, USA

Gleeson Rebello, M.D. Pediatric Orthopedic Surgery, Department of Orthopedics, Mass General Brigham, Boston, MA, USA

Department of Orthopaedic Surgery, Harvard Medical School, Boston, MA, USA

Andrea Reilly, M.D. General Internal Medicine, Department of Medicine, Massachusetts General Hospital, Boston, MA, USA

Department of Medicine, Harvard Medical School, Boston, MA, USA

Department of Pediatrics, Harvard Medical School, Boston, MA, USA

Giuseppina Romano-Clarke, M.D. Newborn Services, Department of Pediatrics, Massachusetts General Hospital, Boston, MA, USA

Department of Pediatrics, Harvard Medical School, Boston, MA, USA

Elizabeth Roux Harvard Medical School, Boston, MA, USA

Emily Silverman, M.D. Department of Medicine, University of California San Francisco, San Francisco, CA, USA

Kathy May Tran, M.D. General Internal Medicine, Department of Medicine, Massachusetts General Hospital, Boston, MA, USA

Department of Medicine, Harvard Medical School, Boston, MA, USA

Bernard E. Trappey, M.D. Center for the Art of Medicine, University of Minnesota Medical School, Minneapolis, MN, USA

Medicine-Pediatrics Hospital Medicine, Department of Medicine and Pediatrics, University of Minnesota Medical School, Minneapolis, MN, USA

Maria Trent, M.D., M.P.H. Adolescent and Young Adult Medicine, Johns Hopkins Children's Center, Baltimore, MD, USA

Department of Pediatrics, Johns Hopkins Medicine, Baltimore, MD, USA

Mai Uchida, M.D. Child Psychiatry Service, Department of Psychiatry, Massachusetts General Hospital, Boston, MA, USA

Department of Psychiatry, Harvard Medical School, Boston, MA, USA

Vinayak Venkataraman, M.D. Sarcoma Center, Department of Medical Oncology, Dana-Farber Cancer Institute, Boston, MA, USA

Department of Medicine, Brigham and Women's Hospital, Boston, MA, USA

Department of Medicine, Harvard Medical School, Boston, MA, USA

Chi T. Viet, D.D.S., M.D., Ph.D. Department of Oral and Maxillofacial Surgery, Loma Linda University Health, Loma Linda, CA, USA

Marc S. Weinberg, M.D., Ph.D. Memory Disorders, Department of Neurology, Massachusetts General Hospital, Boston, MA, USA

Department of Psychiatry, Massachusetts General Hospital, Boston, MA, USA

Department of Psychiatry, Harvard Medical School, Boston, MA, USA

Learning and Training

1

Mark Allan Goldstein, Bernard E. Trappey, Megan Marshall, Shan W. Liu, Trisha K. Paul, Victor A. Lopez-Carmen, and Minali Nigam

M. A. Goldstein (✉)
Adolescent and Young Adult Medicine, Department of Pediatrics, Massachusetts General Hospital, Boston, MA, USA

Department of Pediatrics, Harvard Medical School, Boston, MA, USA
e-mail: mgoldstein@mgh.harvard.edu

B. E. Trappey
Center for the Art of Medicine, University of Minnesota Medical School, Minneapolis, MN, USA

Medicine-Pediatrics Hospital Medicine, Department of Medicine and Pediatrics, University of Minnesota Medical School, Minneapolis, MN, USA

M. Marshall
Medicine-Pediatrics Residency Program, Massachusetts General Hospital, Boston, MA, USA

S. W. Liu
Department of Emergency Medicine, Massachusetts General Hospital, Boston, MA, USA

Department of Emergency Medicine, Harvard Medical School, Boston, MA, USA

T. K. Paul
Quality of Life and Palliative Care, Department of Oncology, St. Jude Children's Research Hospital, Memphis, TN, USA

Department of Hematology, St. Jude Children's Research Hospital, Memphis, TN, USA

V. A. Lopez-Carmen
Medical School, Boston, MA, USA

M. Nigam
Neurology Residency Program, Brigham and Women's Hospital, Boston, MA, USA

Neurology Residency Program, Massachusetts General Hospital, Boston, MA, USA

© The Author(s), under exclusive license to Springer Nature Switzerland AG 2024
M. A. Goldstein, K. M. Tran (eds.), *Becoming a Better Physician*,
https://doi.org/10.1007/978-3-031-69413-4_1

Commentary: Thawing

Bernard E. Trappey

It was mid-April, but a thick blanket of snow had fallen in the hours since I had held her hand and told her that she was dying.

The pathology had resulted late the previous evening. The pancreatic mass seen on her admission CT scan was, as we'd feared, adenocarcinoma. The enlarged lymph nodes in her mesentery and the spots in her lungs meant that it was already at an advanced stage.

Her skin had been cool. Her hand had shaken in mine. The sadness in the room had been overwhelming, and the list of tasks still to be completed before I could escape the hospital for a few hours had hammered incessantly inside my mind. I told her that we would talk more the next day after the oncology team had a chance to see her, and then I had left her and her family to their grief.

A few hours later, I was back at the hospital. I paused in front of a window on the sixth floor of the hospital to answer a phone call. Gray clouds hugged the Mississippi River below. The trees that lined its banks sagged under their burden of heavy, wet, spring snow. It seemed like at any moment they could break from the burden they bore.

The oncology fellow was on the other side of the call. He and his attending had already seen my patient. They had told her that she would only be a candidate for palliative chemotherapy, and that she could expect to live another two to three months at best.

I hung up with a sigh and made my way to her room.

I had put off seeing her that morning. I'd told myself that I had nothing to add until we had a plan from oncology. But, really, I had been avoiding the sadness that I knew would be waiting for me in the room.

But now I had no excuse.

At her door, I rolled my shoulders against the weight of my lab coat. After three years of residency, its once pristine whiteness had become a dingy grayish yellow.

I knocked and announced myself before entering.

I found her husband and seven children crowded around her. Every one of them was smiling—my patient most of all.

"You just missed the oncologists," she said.

"They just called me…" I paused wondering if the oncologists had neglected to tell her the full truth about her situation.

"He said I have three months to live!"

"That's what he told me," I replied, finding myself increasingly untethered from her reality.

"Not weeks!" she said. "Months! I can plant my garden and sit on the porch in the sun and eat pineapple! I get to see another summer!"

From my seat at the edge of her bed, she was framed by the window. Outside, the clouds were beginning to break up, and the landscape seemed a little less bleak. The trees, still bent by the weight of the snow, seemed less likely to break.

She reached for my hand again.

This time, her grip was strong and steady.

And I didn't let go.

Even as she and her family transitioned to talk about the logistics required to get her home.

Even as my pager buzzed.

Even as my attending texted to see if I was ready to round.

This time, I stayed exactly where I needed to be.

That long winter ended eventually, as do all seasons.

I am now a hospitalist at the same academic medical center and have the privilege of working alongside trainees of all levels, and to witness and walk beside them in the long slog of training. Though it has only been a dozen years since I finished training, duty hours and shift structures have changed incrementally but significantly in those years. Still, trainees often seem to spend the majority of their training primarily in survival mode. When I see residents struggle within the current system, it is tempting to turn to stories of how much worse things were "back in my day."

But when I reflect now on my own time in training, the memories of the difficult parts are surprisingly vague and nebulous. I remember the sacrifices I made, the long hours and sleepless nights, the shocking lack of supervision, and the mistakes made. But the sharp edges of anxiety, fatigue, isolation, and loss seem to have been sanded down by the passage of time. However, the lessons I learned and the people from whom I learned them—the mentors, the coworkers, and, most importantly, the patients—remain vivid and alive in my memory.

Yet, no matter how much the rules of medical training may change, the challenges and struggles faced by trainees are universal and immutable. Fortunately, so are the rewards. So, as mentors and role models, instead of minimizing the struggles, we should encourage trainees to lean into the parts of the learning process that bring them some small measure of joy so that the horizon may be illuminated when the days become long and dark.

> Dr. Trappey is a Med-Peds Hospitalist. He is a Co-Director of the Center for the Art of Medicine at the University of Minnesota Medical School. In this role, he is able to pursue his passion for understanding and appreciating the stories that lie at the heart of the practice of medicine and helping medical trainees and professionals become more effective storytellers and artists of all types.

Good Grief

Megan Marshall

As a young child, I was deemed sensitive by some unspoken standard of human disposition. I was quick to cry if I saw another child get hurt—and I was beside myself if there was *any* chance that I had contributed to that hurt. "Sensitive" is how this usually gets labeled. While I didn't necessarily see this as a negative growing up, it was definitely not something I felt proud of. In my experiences thus far in medicine, sensitivity has not been sold as a strength. If I am being honest, entering medical school and even residency, I wondered if my sensitivity would be my downfall. Would my soft heart be able to tolerate witnessing so much suffering? Would I not be overwhelmed by the hurt? I worried constantly.

I tried to prepare myself, considering all possibilities. Students and doctors above me would warn of the stress and anxiety from training and the imposter syndrome that may rise to the surface. There were discussions of coping with anger and frustration toward patients, and even toward colleagues. They spoke of the fear, excitement, and satisfaction yet to come. It was clear to me that despite a long-standing collective yearning for cool, calm, and collected clinical distance, this was emotional work. I only hoped I could persist, despite my sensitive nature.

It was only later, a few years into medical school, when I came across an emotion I couldn't quite identify, that I realized something crucial had been omitted from the forewarnings of the possible emotions I might encounter in my medical practice.

During my clerkship year, I took care of a young woman with lupus. I participated in her care in short bursts—witnessing small snippets of her life, as well as her decline. The first time we met, she was on a surgical service for wound dehiscence following a laparotomy for bowel rupture. She was 31-years-old, charming, warm, and always smiling. She greeted us each day, "Good morning, doctors!" and despite severe pain, she sent us on our way with more enthusiasm than most can muster at such an early hour. "I hope you have a wonderful day!"

A year later, I learned that she was once again admitted to the hospital, and I paid her a visit. So much had changed in a year. She was dependent on a ventilator through a tracheostomy and unable to move unassisted. Despite her worsening condition, her greeting held the same enthusiasm as it had a year before. "How are you doing? I love your shirt!" This time, she mouthed the words, having lost any real use of her voice.

Some months later, I saw her one last time. She was in the intensive care unit, comatose, in multi-organ failure, her body heavy and overwhelmed with fluid. Her family was praying at her bedside. It was the only time I saw her without a smile. She died shortly thereafter. Her death, or rather the loss of her life, brought a tightness in my chest that was hard to shake.

I thought of her often, and eventually I had an opportunity to share this story during a reflection group composed mostly of senior physicians. Tears welled up in my eyes as I fondly remembered my patient and shared the story of our time together. Toward the end of the hour-long session, one of the doctors in the group spoke, "If I were in your shoes, as a medical student, I imagine this might be the first patient for whom I have truly grieved."

There is a quote by poet Mark Nepo that reads, "If pulled, grief is a thread that will leave us naked in song." In that moment, hearing the word "grief" spoken by an experienced, respected physician, allowed me the freedom to pull that thread without hesitation. Now, I find myself scanning the seams for the next thread to pull—eager to see how each new song revealed will guide me through my days.

Sometimes I am caught off-guard. I find myself surprised by the grief I feel for a patient with whom I have only spent a short amount of time. My first instinct (likely influenced by the tradition and reverence of clinical distance) is to feel that I have no right to grieve for them—that the loss is not mine; it belongs to the patient and their loved ones. But then I think again: How many times do I need to see a patient before their loss becomes mine? Is there a concrete threshold? How many minutes must I spend talking to their family, learning about their goals and dreams before I really feel the magnitude of the loss? Over the years, I have found that for me this threshold is variable and impossible to predict. It can be ten minutes, three weeks, or one year. Some patients can leave their mark with just a few words—gifted at connecting, drawing you into their world.

Over time, I have created a ritual to help me remember and cope with the heavier losses. If a patient's loss feels big, I find a physical charm—a symbol of who they were and add it to a silver chain. My silver chain includes a charm for the loss of the melodies sung by my patient with interstitial lung disease (on the few days he was strong enough to walk through the halls of our medical floor). Another for the loss of mobility for my 70-year-old patient who had recently hiked 500 miles before falling ill. There is a Statue of Liberty charm to remind me of a 20-year-old patient who wanted desperately to visit New York City with her mother, but instead was stuck on the pediatric ward for months on end. I'm still searching for the right charm to represent the loss of the curious, bright mind of an elderly woman with a failing heart, who, in her final days before she slipped away, asked me about the mechanism of action of her medication—"just out of curiosity."

I hold this chain in my hand when I start to feel the weight of medical training, the weight of suffering, becoming a little too heavy. I can think of the bright spots—memories of warm smiles, hands held, and stories told. Life is beautiful, and worth grieving.

Unsolicited advice usually falls on deaf ears, so instead I will simply share with you the advice that I give to myself each time I feel grief starting to swell:

Let it swell. Sit with it. Honor the life lost. Honor the care and attention paid. Honor the love spent, invested in the care of another, and try to remember that your grief is good.

> Dr. Marshall has a long-standing interest in palliative care and recently started working with a palliative care community outreach team in Naggalama, Uganda. She plans to continue global palliative care work and pursue a fellowship in palliative care for both children and adults. Additionally, she has a special interest in caring for patients with sickle cell disease.

The Night I Almost Walked Away from Medicine

Shan W. Liu

I clearly remember the night I almost walked out on my career in medicine.

I was a third-year resident in emergency medicine and had arrived at the hospital ED at 11 p.m., ready to grind through another overnight shift. There was only one attending physician on that night to go along with the senior resident (me) and the junior resident—a skeleton crew for the crush of patients who arrived earlier that night, still waiting, impatiently, to be seen.

Then, a group of paramedics stormed in, steering an 80-year-old woman who had respiratory distress through the maze of patients in our trauma center. Her oxygen saturation hovered in the 70s. I assumed her endotracheal tube was too far in and only ventilating the right lung. I had to find out where the tube was so I could retract it and ventilate the left lung.

I went to order a chest X-ray on my computer, but I couldn't. The department's system was down. Minutes passed, and I worried she would code any minute.

The X-ray technician came by, and I asked her to image the patient with the portable X-ray. She said she couldn't, because I hadn't submitted an order.

Flustered, panicked, I scrambled for a paper form and begged our front-desk coordinator to locate the patient's name card. She was harried, too, with the computer system down but figured out how to get the medical record number and create a card I could ink-stamp on the radiology requisition.

Exasperated, I thrust the form into the X-ray tech's hands.

We got the X-ray. I located the tube, adjusted it, and inflated her left lung. Her oxygen sats began to recover, climbing into a normal range. I admitted her to the ICU.

Then I moved on. I had 40 more patients to see that night.

Sometime just before rounds, the computer system came back up, and we caught up on notes, orders, and results.

We had made it. No one died. I was not only exhausted but also triumphant: We stabilized every patient despite the chaos, overcrowding, and computer system failure.

At 8 a.m., with my shift ending, I slumped into a chair and checked my email. A disturbing trail of messages appeared.

The X-ray technician had complained that I was rude and inappropriate in asking her for an X-ray without an order. Our ED administrator agreed, saying it was never appropriate to be unprofessional.

Instantly, I deflated. We had surmounted enormous challenges and still it wasn't enough. Deflation smoldered into anger. For three years of residency, I had given everything, sacrificing sleep, time with my family, driving myself through 24-hours-on 24 hours-off shifts, staying late to finish my notes—even working once with an IV line in my arm because I didn't want to go home.

Nothing—not illness, not fatigue, not my longing for a normal social life—would stop me from fulfilling my dream.

But now, after all that, I wanted to quit.

That was it. I'm leaving residency, I said to the oncoming attending, who was one of my mentors. As emergency physicians, it seems like we can't win. Consults holler at us, surgeons berate us, admitting teams sneer at us for failing to do a better history—all while 30 patients crowd the waiting room.

Despite all this, I have always kept my cool, never yelling at anyone. To be called unprofessional for urging someone to do an X-ray, with a patient's life on the line, hurt me deeply. I know I wasn't kind to the X-ray tech that night, but I was tired, frustrated, stressed out.

My mentor listened as I spilled this on him that morning. Residency is like water torture, he told me, with small drips over time leading to insanity. I can't recall all that he said to keep me from walking out that morning. But I remember this: He listened to me. He cared.

I'm not proud of how I acted with the tech, but, rewinding the night, I see the larger forces at work. I, like everyone else in the hospital, went into medicine to help people—not to be unkind to colleagues or stripped of all empathy.

But when overcrowding pushes our technical and human resources to the breaking point, it's not hard to see why we snipe at each other. I have been on the receiving end of incivility in the ED, and I know how it feels.

The incident changed my career in more than one way. Because of the kind mentor, I didn't quit that night. I completed my residency and later earned a doctorate in health-services research in part because of this event. I wanted to understand systems and how they lead to errors and adverse events. Perhaps I couldn't control how many patients came into the ED, but I could control the research aspect of my life.

Instead of pointing fingers at people I knew were doing their best, I wanted to fix things at the systemic level that led to breakdowns that sapped morale and put patients at risk.

Unfortunately, in the 20 years since I began this research, the healthcare system has only worsened. Doctors, nurses, and physician assistants are leaving, burned out from COVID-19 and ever-increasing requirements for documentation in the electronic medical record.

Systems-level change is hard, I have learned. But we can control how we as individuals confront the challenges.

I can show up to shifts rested. I can say "no" more often so I have the bandwidth when I do see patients. I can work in medical-education research or advocacy that helps me confront the challenges in medical delivery. I can also find passion projects and hobbies that fuel me to have more empathy and patience in the ED. I can step away when I get frustrated. Sometimes, it takes work to be kind.

I'm far from perfect. This is and will always be a demanding job. Perhaps the biggest lesson I've learned is that to be kind to others, I have to be kind to myself.

> Dr. Liu authored the illustrated children's book *Masked Hero: How Wu Lien-Teh Invented the Mask and Ended an Epidemic*, which depicts the story of how her great-grandfather invented the forerunner of the N95 mask a century ago. She started voice lessons recently to bring more joy to family car trips and host better karaoke parties.

Work on Professionalism

Trisha K. Paul

On a frigid morning in late January, I dropped my tote bag onto the ground in the clinician workroom, glad to feel lighter. It was the kind of Minnesotan day where you could throw a bucket of water in the air, and it would freeze before shattering on the ground.

"I'm so proud of myself for being on time to work," I joked to my co-intern Katie, within earshot of my outpatient preceptor typing at his desk. With eyebrows lifted in pained solidarity, Katie's face mirrored my exhaustion. Neither of us wanted to be general pediatricians; lamenting the tragedy of our resident lives became a pastime.

"So I got written feedback on my evals that I should be more enthusiastic," Katie said. It reminded me of how women are told to smile more.

My preceptor swiveled to face us. "Well, Katie, it's important as part of a workplace for you to be enthusiastic."

"But what do you do if you get the feedback that you're too enthusiastic?" I asked. Attendings had remarked on my excitement, but as dark winter days grew longer, I sputtered. "I probably need to be more enthusiastic in clinic."

"No, Trisha, you just need to work on your professionalism," my preceptor said off-handedly.

My reaction was to burst into laughter. I thought he was joking. Bristled by his word choice—*professionalism*? I was sure it must have been a mistake, a misspeak. But, with nothing playful or regretful in his narrow eyes, his cold rigid stare silenced me.

Being unprofessional is not something we joke about in medicine. From our first moments in white coats, we learn that breaking professionalism is one of the greatest sins. There are obvious violations, like intoxication while caring for patients or scalpel-throwing in an operating room. Far more often, being called out for unprofessionalism is subjective, such as having big, curly, natural hair, or spending too much time playing with a pediatric patient during a clinical encounter.

But my preceptor was not kidding. He hurled his accusation at me on stage before an audience of coworkers. Once outside and offstage, I broke character.

"Did you hear what he said?!" I asked Katie, my voice shrill. Humiliated and enraged, I found my body rebelling against the icy facade I had maintained. I melted into a snot-nosed ruckus. "He has never said anything like that to me. And then this, out of nowhere?" Suspended in disbelief, my thinking was static. I, hysterical.

"Ignore him. You know he probably didn't mean it."

What gave me chills was that I didn't know.

I found my preceptor alone at his desk the next morning.

"You mentioned concerns about professionalism. Can you tell me more about that?"

"You need to show more passion for your work." He sipped his coffee. "You have to improve your performance."

I walked along the Mississippi River that night, glad for the negative-degree wind lashing my cheeks. The flurry of my emotions—shock, disbelief, fury, defeat—blurred my recollections of the afternoon like a shaken snow globe that refused to settle. I stopped feeling my toes first, my fingertips numbing, my body frozen. Not unlike my mind.

I tried to take my preceptor's harsh yet vague words to heart. At first, I reverted to the way I performed as a medical student: eager, curious, and borderline overwrought. I exaggerated my excitement about every clinical encounter and asked questions about their pathologies. I fished for feedback about how to improve my performance. I worried whether professionalism concerns would materialize and jeopardize my path to graduation and onward to fellowship.

I was never again told to work on professionalism, by my preceptor or anyone else. In the wake of his unclear feedback, I worried there were others that felt this way who hadn't said anything to me: How many of those who never erupted in front of me secretly harbored concerns like his?

When we had orientation prior to the start of internship, my program director had cautioned us about the long and dark winter days ahead, reminding the group that the sun always rises. But now, every day felt like an act, trying to appear alive and like myself when I felt nothing like me. Second-guessing and focusing on my performance in front of others took me out of being present.

By the end of winter, a few months after my preceptor mentioned professionalism, I understood that my preceptor and I had both erred. He should have known better than to share feedback in such a hurtful way. And I should have been mindful of how fatigue might affect my professionalism.

Several years later, during the last spring of my residency, I didn't think about the accusation of being unprofessional. I no longer thought of my preceptor in the audience. Now that my audience was made up of only me and my patients and families, I could be authentic in the exam room. I had been accepted into my dream fellowship program, the only place in the country offering combined training in pediatric oncology and hospice and palliative care, which represented everything that I was most passionate about in medicine. On my last oncology rotation as a resident, I saw glimpses of myself as the doctor I hoped to be at the end of training when I cared for a patient that I will call Zara.

Zara was hospitalized the entire month, not uncommon for children with aggressive leukemia. She tricycled around her room as her parents and our team talked about her absolute neutrophil count, which told us whether her bone marrow was recovering from chemotherapy and making infection-fighting cells again. Until that number rose, Zara knew she had to remain in the hospital.

"Better start doing some kind of neutrophil dance," my attending said one day with a shrug. Zara stopped pedaling. Her parents laughed. Every morning after sunrise, it became one of our daily questions to her, "Are you doing a neutrophil dance yet?" Days went by, Zara drawing and watching TV and doing anything other than dancing.

Having spent more years of our lives as dancers than as doctors, my co-resident Phoebe and I decided we as Zara's physicians could learn our own neutrophil dance for her. I had performed as a dancer on stage and as a doctor in an exam room. In caring for Zara, I could bring both to the bedside by dancing for her as a doctor. We practiced choreography created by our attending's pre-teen daughter, who coincidentally had composed a routine to Zara's favorite song. But on show day, our last day of the rotation, Phoebe was sick.

The attending and fellow bobbed as background dancers while I performed our neutrophil dance solo. Zara grinned at me from her hospital bed, her mother clapping her hands, and her father holding a phone in the air to film. I thought about how strange it felt to point my toes and plié in front of my patient and her parents. But my body found nothing odd about it, my head turning to follow my hands, my movements sharp with the beat.

By trying to figure out what it meant to improve my performance, I had stretched into a better version of myself. Receiving difficult feedback challenged me to reimagine the kind of doctor that I wanted to be. Was it unprofessional to perform the neutrophil dance for my patient and her parents? Some might say so, but I didn't think it was. My way of improving my performance was by becoming the kind of doctor that was true to who I am.

I was beginning to understand the undisguised and unscripted doctor I wanted to be. Zara's neutrophils didn't rise overnight, but I repeatedly heard a Japanese proverb in my mind that day: "We're fools whether we dance or not, so we might as well dance." It took weeks, but Zara's bone marrow bounced back.

When the attending, fellow, and I reached the last moves of our performance, we crouched to the ground, then jumped as high as we could as the chorus rang, "*Always had high, high hopes.*" With outstretched arms, we reached beyond the ceiling lights. I knew at that moment that dance was the only kind of performance that I wanted to put on for my patients.

Grappling with my preceptor's negative feedback about professionalism helped me realize that I didn't want my doctoring to feel like an act. Instead, I would find ways to be myself for my patients. As a pediatric oncologist and palliative care physician now, I don't think about playing the part of a doctor anymore. I focus on connecting with my immediate audience—my patients, their family, my coworkers—human to human. I don't question whether I should sing the "No More Chemo" song during the workday, wish a patient happy birthday on a Saturday afternoon, or call a mother who is at home with her dying teen as the sun sets. I'm not sure I would have discovered how to be the doctor that I am today if I never received feedback that challenged my professional identity.

> Dr. Paul is a pediatric oncologist in training and a palliative care physician who is passionate about narrative medicine. She is currently pursuing her Master of Fine Arts degree in Creative Nonfiction through New York University Writer's Workshop in Paris. Dr. Paul loves caring for her little free library, dancing barefoot, and collecting anything made of cork.

My Undeserved Coaches

Victor A. Lopez-Carmen (*Waokiya Mani*)

I started amateur boxing when my medical school's promotions and review board (PRB) hit me with "Monitored Academic Status" for "professionalism concerns" in my third year of medical school. A non-Indigenous faculty member had submitted a report to the PRB that I had tried to prepare a patient presentation in an area reserved for faculty and that I was "aggressive" when told I couldn't be there. I had been using that space the past few days, and so I asked where another space was in the unit that I could use to prepare for a patient presentation instead. I called my advisor to let her know about the situation and that I'd be late. Were these actions seen as aggressive? Later, we found out that hospital security had accidentally granted me badge access to the area, which is how I had been getting inside and what contributed to the confusion.

I had never failed a single clinical exam or course in all of medical school, and now I was branded with "Monitored Academic Status." Sometimes I wonder, if I was more like the majority of students and wasn't a large Mexican-Dakota-Yaqui-Indigenous man, would I have been given the benefit of the doubt? Would the faculty member have empathized with me more because I reminded her of her nephew or son? It's an interesting thought, but I couldn't dwell upon it. They had made their decision.

"Monitored Academic Status" had no formal mechanisms for due process. The powerful PRB was made up of mostly senior faculty, none of whom were Indigenous, with the power to pummel students with various probational statuses, each more muzzling than the next. The more students fought, the older students had warned me, the worse it got for them. "Monitored Academic Status" was one step below formal probation—a status, unlike the one I was punished with, that was visible to residency programs—so I had to keep my head down for the time being. I had two tribal governments with legal teams ready to step in and fight this if I needed, but I placed the bigger picture—helping my Indigenous communities as a future doctor—above temporary colonial inconveniences. My elders taught me this painful skill, which I hope future Indigenous students won't need.

I went to the mandatory assimilation program—I mean, professionalism training program—imposed upon me, and I was assigned a professionalism coach. I also took up boxing. Boxing was as an act of rebellion, something that was productive but done so in my own, wild Indigenous way. I was castigated as aggressive, so why not find a way to take my power and agency back? And, I could channel that toward a good cause. I applied and was selected by Haymakers for Hope, a national nonprofit that hosts USA Boxing-official charity boxing matches. They paired me with a local professional boxing gym, Redline Fight Sports, and provided me with training for five months in preparation for a fight in front of thousands at the MGM Fenway Music Hall. In return, I had to raise at least $10,000 that would be split between Harvard's own Dana-Farber Cancer Institute and a cancer organization of my choosing. I dedicated my fight to a Yaqui relative, ceremonial leader, and traditional artist named Paros Baltazar, who had been fighting cancer and sadly passed away on February 10, 2024. Despite the sport no longer being perceived as the gentleman's affair as it was in the 1940s, even the PRB couldn't stop me from getting in a ring for these causes and identifying myself as a student at their medical school wherever my match was advertised, including in a *Harvard Magazine* article that profiled me and why I was fighting.

Being a warrior is in my Indigenous DNA, and I felt like it was my own spiritual protection from the professionalism coaching the PRB required of me. This was my own way to stay connected to the decolonial spirit, to remember who I am, and who my ancestors were. Every day after clinicals, I would drive to the boxing gym and metaphorically hit Western educational assimilatory practices with each left hook to the heavy bag.

It quickly became clear that in the boxing gym, it didn't matter who you were. It didn't matter if you went to Yale or Harvard or were formerly incarcerated. It didn't matter what your politics were. All that mattered was that you put in the work, respected one another, and were a good teammate. All that mattered was your character. I felt at home, because when I actually go home to my Indigenous communities, these standards are the norm. When my elders hear what medical school I attend, they don't care, but in the best of ways. I love that my people and boxers don't care about titles, prestige, wealth, or connections. That is how I wish medicine could be.

My coach at the gym was a fierce lightweight French-Canadian, retired professional boxer, a kickboxing champion, and a former member of Canada's Olympic boxing team. Throughout the training camp, he became like a father figure to me. In my other life, the professionalism coach my medical school assigned to me was surprisingly growing on me, too.

I didn't think I would enjoy professionalism coaching. There, it felt like it did matter who I was. It felt like I was a failure. It felt like a small piece of what my ancestors went through when they were punished for being different, for being Indigenous and acting Indigenous. For being wild. For being aggressive. It was a huge relief, then, when one of the deans told me my coach was a Black surgeon. A Black man who had come from the South and worked his way up the ranks of a Boston hospital to eventually become a dean himself. A Black man who understood harmful stereotypes and how to be professional without sacrificing one's humanity. He gave me advice based on lived experience that resonated with my lived reality. He became another father figure to me.

Whether I deserved my punishment no longer mattered. It led to one of the greatest honors I experienced in medical school—to have two coaches invested in my success: one was a French-Canadian boxer and one was a Black surgeon from the South. They wanted the best for me in the ring, out of the hospital, out of the ring, and in the hospital. I thank the PRB for leading me to them. They both helped me reach my potential. They both helped me grow. I won my boxing match in front of thousands, my family, and my Tribes. They taught me how to handle conflict, how to remain disciplined, and to always be considerate of teammates, whether in the boxing gym or on the clinical floor.

The struggles of being Indigenous in this world would continue, but medical school became slightly easier and my Indigenous health advocacy partnerships blossomed. I still have much to learn. I am grateful for this journey with my coaches. They are still teaching me how to be a more effective warrior for my people, my patients, and future generations.

> Mr. Lopez-Carmen, an enrolled member of the Crow Creek Sioux Tribe and also from the Yaqui Nation, had ancestral strength instilled in him from the very beginning of life. After receiving his traditional name and baptism as a baby on the Pascua Yaqui Reservation, he attended traditional ceremonies every year of his life and remains an active cultural participant in his communities today. In 2022, he became the first documented Native American to make the Forbes 30 under 30 list in the Healthcare category. In 2024, he made history by becoming the first enrolled member of the Crow Creek Sioux Tribe to graduate from an Ivy League university, and the first male-identifying member to become a physician. He will be pursuing his residency at Seattle Children's Hospital of the University of Washington.

Married in Medicine

Minali Nigam

In my intern year, on my second shift in the cardiac ICU, I received the following page, "The patient's heart rate is in the 160s, please come bedside." Rahul, my senior resident, had stepped out to grab lunch so I was the only doctor on the floor. At the bedside, the telemetry showed wide, mountain-looking peaks that I recognized as ventricular tachycardia. The patient's blood pressure started to fall, as he was decompensating quickly. I called Rahul on the phone and asked him for help. I don't know how he got there so quickly but within a minute he entered the room and knew exactly what to do. He spoke with the nurse, asked for the code cart, and then placed shock pads on the patient. We did anything and everything that we could to get this patient out of V-tach: called a code, gave amiodarone and lidocaine, shocked the patient. We spent hours and hours in this patient's room but the wide peaks on telemetry weren't dissipating.

There was a mix of sadness and frustration about our inability to help the patient. But, at the same time, I was enamored by the way Rahul was doctoring. He seemed calm and collected, even though there was chaos around us. Meanwhile, I was just putting in orders on the computer. My shift ended, and the patient remained in V-tach. Rahul was still in the room, going into the night portion of his 24-hour shift. I learned the next morning that Rahul was able to advocate for the patient's family to come into the hospital. This was peak COVID-19 when visiting policies were restrictive, and we were giving updates to families over the phone. Rahul spoke with the nursing coordinator and made sure the family was able to come in person to say their last goodbyes. I realized then that the senior resident I was working with was an incredibly good, kind person. He saw beyond just caring medically for the patient. My career crush soon turned into an actual crush the more I worked with him and saw interactions between him and our coworkers and patients. On Rahul's last day on service, I gave him a treat basket hoping this would leave a lasting impression. A few days later, on Christmas Eve, I got a text from Rahul, "Hey! It was a blast working with you. Would you want to grab a bite sometime?"

We would find time to meet each other late in the evening, on little sleep in between our work shifts. We would go the extra mile for each other—cooking food or cleaning each other's apartment if one of us had a particularly difficult rotation. There was an ease with Rahul, a feeling of home. We got engaged ten months later, entering a tumultuous time as a couple.

I was in the toughest year of my neurology residency, working frequent 24-hour and night shifts. Rahul was applying for a cardiology fellowship, with the additional stress of trying to match in the same city so we could be together. The little mutual time we had went into wedding planning or attending friends' weddings and family events. We had very limited bandwidth to nurture our relationship, prompting us to take out frustrations with our work schedules on each other. Small disagreements became prolonged and exacerbated as our call shifts made us go 24 to 48 hours without being able to communicate with each other to bring closure.

Medicine is what brought us together, but it was soon becoming the driving force keeping us apart. We both struggled, hanging by a thread, to keep the relationship going. The year came and went with growing pains.

During my working hours as a first-year neurology resident, I constantly had to be "on," being present, performing my best as the most junior resident on the team, while learning and absorbing as much knowledge as I could. There were shifts that were so overwhelming with the number of patients and high level of acuity, that I felt as if I had used all of my cognitive load at work and had very little to give afterward, especially in my personal relationships. Meanwhile, Rahul was finishing up his last year of residency and had matched into a cardiology fellowship in the same city (a huge relief!)—long distance on top of all the stressors on our day to day would have been insurmountable.

We got through the year constantly reminding ourselves of why we chose to be together in the first place: that we shared core values and life goals, that we inspired each other to be a better version of ourselves, and that we loved and respected each other and our families. I focused on the ways Rahul would take care of me, in spite of his busy days, by leaving a glass of water on my nightstand, tucking me in bed when I had a cold, or buying me groceries on a busy rotation. Our communication improved—we would schedule important conversations and try to address issues on the spot, rather than waiting days when our call shifts came in between. On tough days, I had to remind myself of the qualities I admired about Rahul—his intelligence, kindness, and ability to bring people together, among many others.

We got married almost a year after our engagement. Our wedding celebrations felt magical and surreal, surrounded by friends and family from all stages of our lives.

And yet, even post-marriage, our medical training continued, as I was only halfway through residency and Rahul was just starting his fellowship. Weekends together became even more scarce due to Rahul's fellowship demands. As my work schedule started to become lighter, his became the opposite. It felt as if we couldn't catch a break.

We recently had a "golden weekend" in which both of us had Saturday and Sunday off together at home—not traveling or going to events or working at the hospital. We had time to just be together without any plans, a feat that took a year and a half to accomplish.

We remind ourselves that we will get more of this protected time, one day soon, when we are both out of training. We know that we're not alone as a married couple in medicine. We understand that the care and attention we give our patients, we can't always reciprocate to each other. As medical trainees, our jobs can be so physically and cognitively demanding that sometimes quality time means just sitting next to each other on the couch watching TV or sleeping when we come back home.

After one year of marriage, we've learned that nurturing each other and the relationship still takes a lot of work. There are times we get impatient, irritated, or misunderstand each other. There are times when we just need space from each other. But the key for us is knowing that we are a constant support for each other. In a job that is surrounded by suffering, coming home to each other is a form of healing and comfort.

We listen and talk through mistakes while we're on the job without judgment. On tough workdays, simply holding each other's hands is all that's needed to cheer each other up. We share our career ambitions and dreams, looking to each other for guidance as we navigate through our medical training. We learn from each other and, in turn, become better doctors by talking through challenging patient or colleague encounters, sharing the latest research or medical news articles, and actively listening to each other, an important skill we employ when caring for patients.

From my marriage, I have grown into a more empathetic, understanding, and caring physician. I could have never thought that what started as a call shift in the cardiac ICU would turn into a lifetime of doctoring together.

> Dr. Nigam graduated from the University of North Carolina (UNC) School of Medicine and earned a degree from the UNC Hussman School of Media and Journalism. As a physician-journalist, she hopes to share stories that raise public health awareness and make medicine (especially neurology) easier to understand. Outside of medicine, she enjoys yoga, running, swimming, and trying out new restaurants in the Boston area.

Career

2

Kathy May Tran, Michael F. Bierer, Mai Uchida,
Farrin A. Manian, Michelle L. Izmaylov, Erica C. Kaye,
Joseph R. Betancourt, Andrea Reilly, and Michael Jellinek

K. M. Tran (✉) · M. F. Bierer
General Internal Medicine, Department of Medicine, Massachusetts General Hospital, Boston, MA, USA

Department of Medicine, Harvard Medical School, Boston, MA, USA
e-mail: kathy.tran@mgh.harvard.edu

M. Uchida
Child Psychiatry Service, Department of Psychiatry, Massachusetts General Hospital, Boston, MA, USA

Department of Psychiatry, Harvard Medical School, Boston, MA, USA

F. A. Manian
Department of Medicine, Mercy Hospital-St. Louis, St. Louis, MO, USA

Department of Medicine, St. Louis University Medical School, St. Louis, MO, USA

Department of Medicine, Ponce Health Sciences University, St. Louis, MO, USA

M. L. Izmaylov
General Internal Medicine and Public Health, Department of Medicine, Vanderbilt University Medical Center, Nashville, TN, USA

E. C. Kaye
Quality of Life and Palliative Care, Department of Oncology, St. Jude Children's Research Hospital, Memphis, TN, USA

J. R. Betancourt
General Internal Medicine, Department of Medicine, Massachusetts General Hospital, Boston, MA, USA

Department of Medicine, Harvard Medical School, Boston, MA, USA

Commonwealth Fund, New York, NY, USA

A. Reilly
General Internal Medicine, Department of Medicine, Massachusetts General Hospital, Boston, MA, USA

Department of Medicine, Harvard Medical School, Boston, MA, USA

Department of Pediatrics, Harvard Medical School, Boston, MA, USA

M. Jellinek
Child Psychiatry Service, Department of Psychiatry, Massachusetts General Hospital, Boston, MA, USA

Department of Psychiatry, Harvard Medical School, Boston, MA, USA

Department of Pediatrics, Massachusetts General Hospital, Boston, MA, USA

Commentary: My COVID Epitaph

Michael F. Bierer
If I do not survive COVID
Please note the hopes we shaped before
The concerts, hikes and family feasts
Still on schedule, still in store.
I can write my colleagues' tributes now
I hope you will be flattered,
How you toiled, co-authored, supported staff.
You smiled when it mattered.
But we will die. I'm sorry, friend,
That for us it could be
Sharply, while we labor on
Do you think that's as it should be?
In the hallways, exam rooms, and clinics
Doctoring amid pain and tears
Shared mission, on-call nights, holding,
Kind gravitas calming our fears.
What I left of me at the hospital
Created a void we sensed elsewhere
Keying our door, scratching sweet Maggie
In my lap, iPhone, my comfy chair.
They bravely passed with no regrets.
We salute them now
We loved, respected and mourn them
But whom did I fail and how?

> Dr. Bierer is a member of the Addiction Consult Team at Massachusetts General Hospital (MGH) and Brigham and Women's Faulkner Hospital. He has helped teach and coordinate addiction education for medical residents for decades and now also teaches addiction fellows. The challenges of medical training have made him attuned to the struggles of colleagues and motivated him to share in the care of their patients, whose pain and grief they carry. When Dr. Bierer wrote this poem, he was in the inaugural cohort of the Public Voices Fellowship at MGH, recovering from bilobar pneumonia, and the initial wave of a mysterious and high-fatality virus was a looming, dark presence.

Finding Empathy While Fighting Misinformation

Mai Uchida

A few days after New Year's Day in 2021, I became one of the first pregnant women to receive the COVID-19 mRNA vaccine. After weighing the risks of vaccination versus the risks of not getting vaccinated, my decision was crystal clear. I decided for myself, my unborn third son in utero, my family, my patients, and my community. After getting the vaccine, I worked with the outreach groups at the Massachusetts General Hospital (MGH) to share my personal story, as well as the scientific data on vaccination and pregnancy, with the hope that our community would be empowered to make the decision to vaccinate on their own terms. The moment that the media content went viral in my home country of Japan, where there was significant hesitancy toward vaccinations, was the serendipitous event that changed my life.

While it was clear that the overall impact of my communication to the public was very positive, I also received gestures of hate from people who were part of the anti-vaccine movement. I was accused of being a bad mother, because it was "child abuse" to vaccinate as a pregnant mom. MGH and Harvard received anonymous emails about my "unethical conduct" for recommending vaccination to pregnant people. There were Exacto-knife blades that arrived in the physical mail addressed to me. A fake death certificate was made for my unborn baby that declared, "Reason of death: mother's vaccination." The response gradually expanded beyond the topic of vaccination and evolved into comments about my appearance, how I spoke, and about my being a woman. I was reminded of the deep-seeded gender inequalities in the Japanese culture. The thousands of online comments and direct messages kept pouring in.

This unexpected experience made me realize a few things: (1) the power of misinformation in impacting one's health, (2) the lack of support for parents who need to make hard decisions for their families, and (3) the psychological harm of unconscious biases that connect to inequality.

As parents—particularly mothers—we are often put in positions where we need to make responsible decisions for our children, yet it's so hard to access scientific and accurate knowledge that will allow us to make those decisions. In addition, we are rarely given support to walk through that process, and we are somehow always criticized for the decisions we make for our children, no matter what decision that might be.

This was very familiar to me both as a mother and a child psychiatrist. Unfortunately, child psychiatry has been a field of abundant misinformation and prejudice. While theories that mothers who act "cold" could "create" children with autism or psychosis have been scientifically debunked many decades ago, the terms "refrigerator mothers" and "schizophrenogenic mothers" still continue to be used in some circles. Parents of children who struggle psychiatrically are often shamed and made to feel guilty. Even the existence of pediatric mood disorders that have neurobiological underpinnings, such as depression or bipolar disorder, continue to be a topic of dispute, and parents continue to be blamed for their children's mood dysregulations. There are various treatments that could help children and families with social and emotional difficulties, but misinformation and prejudice create a high barrier for the people who need help to seek it out.

Misinformation and prejudice can significantly alter or even end lives. To tackle misinformation and prejudice, we need to advance science and disseminate knowledge. I made a pledge a long time ago that this would be part of my life's work. Being a child psychiatrist, never in my life had I imagined that it would happen in this way, as I became a scientific advocate during an infectious disease pandemic. When the world was suffering, however, I knew that I had to carry out my pledge.

When I received the overwhelming amount of hate from those who were hesitant about vaccinating, I took a deep breath, hugged my family, gathered my support system, and decided to talk to the "haters." I went onto Japanese national TV every single day for more than half a year and spoke from my heart.

As a clinician-researcher, I thoughtfully explained the scientific evidence of the mRNA vaccine and clinical data on COVID-19. I did so with empathy and understanding of the struggles of the pandemic, as well as the fear that people felt toward the vaccine. I discussed the risks and benefits of vaccination, and I spoke about my own hardships of being a mother of three as the world shut down. I was eventually asked to join a nonprofit project founded by like-minded doctors to tackle medical misinformation surrounding the COVID-19 vaccine. Together, we worked with the media and the Japanese government in delivering accurate scientific information to the public.

Thankfully, people listened. In January 2021, only 7% of the Japanese population responded that they planned to receive the COVID-19 vaccine. By September 2021, over 80% had already received at least two doses of the vaccine. In 2022, our nonprofit received the Minister of Health, Labour and Welfare Award, which is given to medical advocates that made the most health impact in Japan.

I also had a hidden agenda of feminism throughout this mission. As I mentioned, many of the comments that I personally received during the vaccine advocacy targeted the fact that I was a woman. The World Economic Forum ranks Japan 125th out of 149 countries in gender equality. In my Japanese medical school class that graduated in 2007, there were only 15 women out of 100 students. My male classmates frequently stated with confidence that they did not think that women should become doctors. In 2018, an investigation found that multiple medical schools in Japan systematically deducted female applicants' scores on entrance exams to reduce the number of female doctors. Their inexcusable justification was because "women have children and can't work as much as men." This statement was widely accepted by the public. My decision to leave Japan was directly related to systematic sexism.

When I started appearing on Japanese national TV for vaccine advocacy, it was a shock to the viewers. Not only had I been vaccinated as a pregnant person but also I was a female physician in a leadership position at Harvard, while having a family. This incited microaggressions such as, "I initially doubted you because I thought you are a woman who has 'won' it all," to comments that sexualized or attacked me directly. I, of course, did not enjoy these statements, but it made it clear that there is a need for representation of women with expertise. I felt even more that I needed to be present in the media and have these academic conversations, and so I continued to talk publicly about my experiences as a Japanese female physician and why systematic sexism is a problem for both men and women.

Throughout this experience, I had many conversations with people who were on the other side. Initially, I assumed that there was a separation of "us" and "them." What opened my eyes was that many of the people who showed hesitancy about the vaccine shared the same goal as people who advocated for vaccination: to protect the health of ourselves and our loved ones.

I will carry this lesson with me, as I live through a time in American history when the divisions of society are undeniable. In the past, I used to think about divisions of ideologies as two colors never mixing together, separated by a clear line. I used to envision "crossing the divide" as changing the entire color of the other side. Finding empathy for people who appeared to be on the opposite side allowed me to think differently. Now I realize that the colors and divisions are much more nuanced. There is a gradation of each color from dark to light, and there are parts where two colors mix. "Bridging the divide" might mean that we are able to cherish the nuances of the colors, even to change the tones of those colors on divisive issues.

> Dr. Uchida is a mother of three sons, a pediatric psychiatrist, a neuroscience researcher, and an internationally acclaimed advocate for mental health, scientific literacy, and gender equality. During the COVID-19 pandemic, Dr. Uchida made significant impact as a scientific communicator addressing the strong vaccine hesitancy in Japan. She is the author of four books *Social Justice, Reappraisal, Prescriptions for Everyday Mental Crises,* and *Living Depression: A Conversation Between a Psychiatrist and a Patient.*

No Silence, Please!

Farrin A. Manian

As I hastily scroll through the newsfeed on my dimly lit tablet screen and try not to doze off in the late night, one headline stops me in my tracks: "Healthcare workers being fired because of speaking out against their employers." Now wide awake,

I begin reading the content of the article, not just out of curiosity as a healthcare worker, but with a sense of genuine empathy for fired physicians dating back to my own experience some 25 years ago. Although I prefer not to dwell on that turbulent chapter in my life, I find myself revisiting it more often than I wish, thanks in large part to today's healthcare climate.

That fateful Tuesday morning was the day after the Labor Day holiday. I had just returned to work after a much-needed three-day weekend break and, as might be expected, I was busy rounding on my hospital patients trying to catch up on all the events that had transpired in my absence. Much less expected was a call from the CEO's office asking me to meet with him urgently to discuss my contract. This was an odd request because my contract with the hospital, where I had worked as an infectious disease physician for over 10 years, had recently been updated following the merger of the hospital with a larger healthcare system. Without much delay, I interrupted my rounds and headed toward the CEO's office. After taking a seat outside his office door for what felt like an eternity, the CEO finally emerged. As he shut the door behind me, he delivered the shocking news: "Your contract has a no-cause clause in it and it's going to be terminated." "You keep writing about us!" he added grudgingly.

The CEO was referring to my recent articles on the state of healthcare in this country based on my experiences as a practicing physician. In my first article, "Should We Accept Mediocrity?" published in the *New England Journal of Medicine* in April 1998, I discussed what I referred to as "DEFs" or "deficiencies, errors, and frustrations" that I had observed in the course of my practice when navigating a healthcare system that seemed to turn a deaf ear to physicians' concerns and, in some respects, gravitated toward accepting mediocrity as a new normal. The article resonated with many of my fellow physicians locally and nationally who often felt unheard as they, too, tried to navigate new systems of healthcare that seemed to jeopardize patient safety. Some physician leaders with administrative positions at my institution, however, were less congratulatory and felt that my concerns were best shared internally, not publicly, even though I never mentioned the name of my employer in my writing.

A subsequent piece, "Whither Continuity of Care?" published in the *New England Journal of Medicine* in September 1999, was prompted by a new national trend—present even today—toward fragmentation of healthcare delivery and the diminishing role of the primary care physician (once regarded as the "captain of the ship") in coordinating patient care. Among many concerns, I questioned the merits of discouraging competent internists from caring for their hospitalized patients as a means of increasing their office practice productivity. As before, the article was well-received by many of my colleagues locally and afar who took the time to call me, drop me a line, or even walk over to my office just to shake my hand. One cardiology colleague even rushed into my office, jumping up and down in jubilation as if celebrating the defeat of Goliath at the hands of David. In contrast, some of the local physician leaders who were tasked with implementation of new systems of care were less than complimentary. They felt that change should be embraced and that my writings served very little purpose other than undermine the reputation of my employer, even though, again, I never mentioned the hospital by name. Unfortunately, my long-lasting friendships with those physicians was adversely affected and, as a result, I lost a few friends. It became clear to me that the changes in our healthcare system was increasingly pitting physicians against physicians, which then prompted me to write another perspective article on the same subject in the *Archives of Internal Medicine* in March 2001.

The writing piece that appeared to seal my fate, however, was a counterpoint editorial that I had written in response to a commentary in the local newspaper by a hospital association executive. In his editorial, the executive attempted to dissuade the nurses from unionization in local hospitals and implored them to remain loyal to hospital leaders as members of a large family to resolve their differences. Without mentioning the name of any hospital, I felt that for nurses to remain loyal to their employers, their concerns about salaries and new systems of patient care needed to be taken seriously by the C-suite. Asking healthcare workers to make concessions while ignoring their demands defied logic and further incentivized them to unionize, I argued. The CEO was visibly upset with me for expressing my views on the subject in the local newspaper, and he even suggested that the main reason I wrote about healthcare topics was to bring attention to myself, not the healthcare issues that mattered to me. I was shocked and hurt by this baseless accusation.

After a long and contentious exchange of words, it became increasingly clear to me that further attempts to convince the CEO to reconsider my dismissal would be futile. Baffled and indignant, I got up out of my chair and left his office without saying another word. "How can I—in a country known around the world as the beacon of individual freedom and where the first amendment of its constitution guarantees free speech—be summarily terminated for publicly expressing my views on healthcare matters that affect patients everywhere?" I asked myself. I was convinced that the CEO had overstepped his authority and had no right terminating my contract for speaking out.

Of course, I was wrong! By the next day, I found out that most states have "employment-at-will" statutes which allow employers to dismiss employees without a stated cause. In addition, my friends in the legal profession were quick to remind me that the freedom of speech rights in this country only apply to the U.S. government as it deals with its citizens, not to private employers when dealing with their employees. Clearly, I underestimated the power of employers to fire their employees without cause and the limitations of the right to free speech under the first amendment.

Over the ensuing days, the news of my dismissal spread like wildfire throughout the hospital with many of my colleagues and coworkers openly expressing their dismay with the leadership's decision. A petition for a vote of no-confidence in the CEO soon began to circulate among hospital staff demanding that the administration reverse its decision. As emotionally and physically draining that the ordeal was for me and my family, I was honored and deeply touched by the level of support and validation that I received from the staff. After two weeks of hospital-wide vocal opposition, the CEO informed me that my termination letter has been rescinded and that I could continue to work under the terms of my recent contract, as if nothing had happened. I thanked him for the offer, but I let him know that I had learned my lesson and could no longer accept the terms of my contract as written. Specifically, I demanded that it be amended to recognize my right to engage in public discourse of healthcare issues that mattered to me as a physician—a right that I naively thought I had for years but never did. "I have lost seven pounds in the last two weeks and have gained nothing but the realization that I can get fired anytime because of my writings," I said to the CEO. He balked at my demand. A stalemate ensued.

The news of my dispute with the hospital administration over the freedom of speech clause soon led to a packed meeting hall of hundreds of physicians on staff formally denouncing the actions of the administration. Not long after, the local medical society and the news media joined the action. A front-page Sunday morning article in the local paper about physicians losing their jobs for speaking out particularly struck a chord with the public. Rapid-fire coverage by local radio and television stations and newspapers, including letters to the editor by many of my then current and former patients denouncing hospital executives for trying to control the narrative of their physician employees eventually led to an amendment to my contract. More specifically, the amendment granted me the freedom to speak out as long I refrained from making inaccurate, incomplete, libelous, or defamatory statements against my employer, something that I had never done or planned to do. In fact, I did not participate in any of the staff's gatherings voicing opposition to my termination and declined interviews by the news media throughout the entire tumult. I simply did not wish to serve as a distraction from the basic principle of the right to free speech that I felt all physicians should have.

After carefully reading the entire article, I set the tablet down on my nightstand. I close my eyes, but I am still wide awake, asking the same questions I asked 25 years ago: Will doctors be free to share their experience publicly and express their views on healthcare matters without fear of retribution by their employers? Will periodic news of physicians losing their jobs for speaking out serve as a reminder of the potential price of insubordination and discourage others from doing the same? Will physicians be forced to choose between job security and advocacy for the welfare of their patients? And, if they don't speak out when they should, will the medical profession risk losing the trust of the public? With an increasing number of physicians becoming employees of larger healthcare entities, the answers to these and similar questions are even more relevant today than they were a quarter century ago.

I muse over how, early in my career, it was common for hospitals to post signs of "Be quiet" or "Silence, please" on the wards in hopes of helping sick patients heal by reducing noise. I believe today's healthcare organizations should actively promote a seemingly contradictory policy of "No silence, please" among their physician employees when it comes to expression of concerns over practices that might adversely impact patient care. Patient care and physician morale are sure to improve.

Perhaps, Reverend Martin Luther King said it best: "Our lives begin to end the day we become silent about things that matter."

I had a hard time falling asleep that night.

> Dr. Manian is an infectious diseases physician who turned academic hospitalist over a decade ago to become more closely involved in the education of medical students and residents during their formative years of training. He is a strong proponent of "writing to learn" and is the editor of *www.pearls4peers.com*, an open-access, free educational website based on clinical questions raised during patient rounds. He is an amateur photographer (*www.doctorsbestshots.com*) and even a more amateur gardener.

Instead of That Phone Call

Michelle L. Izmaylov

On an admitting shift, I place a consult asking for a specialist to assess a patient. He calls back quickly. I have already received ten calls today, and I ask whether we can text instead.

Several hours later, I am walking to my car when I encounter the consultant in a hallway. He steps between me and the elevator, his body obscuring the door behind him. I step back when he approaches. The consultant demands to know why I asked to text instead of calling. He tells me: *Everyone prefers phone calls to texting.* The consultant is prepared with his reasons—that it is easier and more professional—speaking with the certainty of a textbook. My body bends beneath those words, even my ribs folding like a fan, without interruption or resistance to his argument.

He walks away, and I feel small standing in that hallway, wondering the words I do not speak out loud to the consultant: *Am I the only one who prefers texting to phone calls?*

This scenario unfolds many times on any given shift. I am quick to answer each text message, wanting to respond to what my colleagues need. But when there's an incoming phone call, I look at the screen for a while, steadying myself before picking up the phone. Sometimes there are many phone calls within several minutes, a list of colleagues to call back, my anxiety increasing with every call that I have to make. I know what might happen when they pick up the phone, pepper me with a series of questions to which I might not have the answers, followed by the groan of irritation when I ask for a chance to collect data and then text back with the information that is needed, not meeting their expectation that everyone should be skilled at quickly providing every necessary piece of information over a phone call.

Maybe it is only me who needs the moment offered by texting to collect my thoughts, the moment to express what I would like to communicate better than I could through spoken conversation. Over a phone call, I would tell you there is a patient who would like to ask the gastroenterology specialist a question. In text, I can tell you of the cascade of fire that is the patient's hair as she sits in a chair, her shoulders not slumped beneath the news we have brought her of the endoscopy showing inflammatory bowel disease, but instead her hands gathering up the words for her diagnosis and the medications we have prescribed, determined to overcome this.

I know that tone and body language speak more than the words we say. Sometimes I am overwhelmed, with many patients to see on rounds and a rapid response to run to. I ask you to allow me to conceal those emotions, to communicate the information you are asking for in words without the anxiety that would be apparent in my voice. I am not always prepared to pretend that I am fine at every moment, as I must do on the phone. Rather, in a text, I can tell you my intended message without revealing what I would not like you to know, and then I can have the moment I need for my emotions to settle.

Texting offers me another aspect of protection. The words I say out loud are small, not nearly strong enough to deflect an argument, and I fold at the slightest pressure. In text, I can organize my own argument and consider what you are asking for without the pressure of providing an immediate response. Is this not better than for me to agree with your every statement, only for you to walk away while I stand holding the words that I wanted to tell you?

Maybe in my preference, there is weakness, but there is also a certain strength. Perhaps not everyone would see the good in this, but there are benefits I have noticed.

My voice is not the loudest in the room and is not usually the first to be heard. Because of that, I hear my patient's voice instead, allowing their words to fill up the room instead of mine. As an intern, a patient presents with too much fluid gathered in her legs. I listen while she talks about her cats, telling me about the food they like and the stores where that food is available. She buys the best food for her cats, saving up her money. The patient tells me of her trip to the store this week, how she walked past the vegetables, not even glancing at the prices she could not afford. She buys canned food for herself, buying better food for her cats. I listen and I learn what she does not tell me directly, that she eats more sodium than she should because those are the foods she can afford.

At a crowded event, I am most often found by the walls and away from the commotion. I am not the center of attention, but from my position, I notice others who have been pushed to the periphery. As a senior resident, I notice the intern who stands in a corner holding her fifth alcoholic drink, the intern I later find vomiting in the parking lot of the event venue. She has another ICU shift tomorrow. I listen while she tells me how these past few months have felt like stones tied around her body. We watch a car moving across the parking lot. She tells me that, if that car were coming at her, she is not certain that she would want to move.

I consult social work to provide the patient with food resources, and I walk with the intern to the employee assistance program office where she seeks help for burnout. My voice might not be the loudest, but I strive for my ears to hear what you would really need to say, for my eyes to see what you would really need me to notice, and when you tell me that everyone prefers phone calls to texting, I wonder if you even see that I am standing there in front of you.

My colleagues occasionally complain that I do not communicate. But there is something not included when they express their concerns. Maybe I do not like to communicate in the manner that they demand, a manner that does not consider my own concerns at having another phone call to answer, that does not account for my own preference for expressing thoughts. Does communication only count when it is performed over a phone call? Is it necessary to prefer phone calls to be a good physician?

Maybe instead of the argument in a hallway, maybe instead of the assumptions and the words that hurt—the words that make those like me wonder whether we have a place in medicine—we could each communicate in the way that we prefer.

I have asked colleagues whether I can text instead of calling about patients. There are many who do not agree. But I sometimes get a glimpse of how things could be—the consultant who asks whether I would prefer to text, the colleague who agrees to try what I am asking for. With each request, I work to help more people understand that not everyone shares any certain preference. Even when we agree on a phone call, when I allow your preference to override my own, I ask that you recognize an action that comes from my respect for you. We do it your way for this patient. Then we could try my way for the next patient.

Maybe many people prefer a phone call.

But the voices of those who prefer to speak through text have value, too.

> Dr. Izmaylov is a first-generation American whose narrative medicine essays have been widely published, including in *The Lancet Psychiatry* and *Annals of Internal Medicine*. She is an advocate for clinician well-being and has presented on narrative medicine at grand rounds across the country.

Hard Work

Erica C. Kaye

When I receive an invitation to a mandatory "work–life balance" panel, I mark the date on my calendar with care. As a trainee, I've grown accustomed to arriving at the hospital at dawn and leaving at midnight. My life is a revolving door of work with no pretense of balance, and I am anxious to find strategies to help reset my equilibrium.

On the day of the session, I arrive early and sit in the first row. A panel of five faculty, four men and one woman, sit behind a table at the front of the room. The men are smiling, leaning back in their chairs, chatting comfortably with each other. The woman sits quietly, poker-faced, detached from their camaraderie.

The panel begins. Each man, in turn, tells his story about finding "work–life balance." From junior and mid-career to senior faculty, they talk about a passion for science and the need to "buckle down" and invest time in the work. Our facilitator lobs a softball: "Can you have a successful career and also prioritize family?" "Of course!" they laugh, reassuringly. A senior faculty reaches for the microphone: "I'm a living example of how you can succeed in research and in your home life, if you're willing to work hard. I'm at the hospital by 6 a.m. each day, I put my nose to the grindstone, and I always come home by 6 p.m. to have dinner with the kids."

Murmurs of approval rustle in the audience. I shift in my seat, accidentally catching the eye of the woman. The panel seems to notice her, too, and they pass the microphone magnanimously down the line. She holds the microphone with both hands, as if it were heavy. "I don't have a partner or children," she says. "So I guess I have it easy?" She pauses, and her question floats in the air, unanswered. "I try to find balance in my personal life…but it is…hard."

The room is silent for an awkward moment. Then the senior faculty, his voice cheerful, plucks the microphone back: "Yes! Absolutely. It *is* hard. But those who work hard enough can have it all." He smiles knowingly, arms crossed in satisfaction over his chest, as he nods to his audience. We clap politely and file out, running back to the hospital wards to catch up on our clinical duties.

I go through the motions of admitting patients, running to emergencies, writing notes. I feel unnerved and unable to concentrate. I tell myself that I'm embarrassed for the woman and her clumsy disclosure of weakness. But beneath my discomfiture, I'm also angry. I feel like her failure, by extension, taints the reputation of women in general. My face burns, remembering the judgment on the other panelists' faces. I am determined to stake out a grindstone, apply my nose, and prove that I, too, can have it all.

I work myself to the bone. Long hours, head down, no time to pause. I tell myself that I just need to make it through training. I just need to get that grant, to publish those papers, to get promoted. I scramble for childcare, work through weekends, cram in late nights. I can have it all. I can work hard and come home for dinner with the kids. *Just like them.*

I join faculty and become the exhausted mother of three young children. My partner is also a full-time physician-scientist. I "balance" clinical, research, education, and leadership responsibilities. On paper, it looks like I've made it.

But what does "making it" look like? I see patients on a busy clinical service, while also trying to submit a massive grant by the deadline. I get a call that my kid is vomiting and needs to be picked up from daycare. My partner is covering his service, without backup. I scramble to find someone to cover me for an hour, so I can drive to daycare, bring the kid home, and make a dozen phone calls to find a last-minute sitter. When the sitter arrives, I return to the hospital, finish seeing patients, and pick up the remaining children from aftercare. Power through dinner, bath, and bedtime. Do three loads of vomit-soaked laundry, pack lunches and backpacks, make another round of calls to find childcare for the next day. Realize that summer camp deadlines are tomorrow, register the kids in the last minute, research hypoallergic sunscreens, buy multiple brands to test out in the coming week. Write consult and progress notes. At midnight, I finally start working on the grant.

I see my work–life "balance" reflected in the haggard faces of my female colleagues. We are working hard, unmistakably, yet little of the work is seen or valued. There is a constant churning of legs under water, with a focus on minimizing ripples. We hemorrhage energy into keeping the surface placid—"proof" that we can cut it.

Subconsciously, I begin to catalogue the labor of the women around me. I observe how we surreptitiously wipe away the sweat on our foreheads as we sprint in place. I watch us get passed over for mentorship and sponsorship, rejected for promotion, pushed out of the ivory tower. We rarely mention the missingness, the holes in our community. But the drip, drip, drip of attrition is loud, like rain on a tin roof, inside my head.

Unspoken questions slowly spill over. Why did she leave academic medicine? Was the work "too hard" for her to handle? Or was work–life balance an empty promise, a rug ripped out from under her feet, with no safety rails in reach? Maybe she recognized a fatal malalignment between the system and her values, and she opted to leave with dignity?

No, I hear, a dozen different ways. She didn't succeed because she failed to publish enough high-impact papers. She wasn't "cut out" for the grind. She wasn't a "good sport." She didn't "lift up" her team. Not everyone can handle the "hard work."

Some days, I imagine myself running on a treadmill, at a 15-degree incline. The floor accelerates under me at a cutthroat, intransigent pace, and I gallop to stay within reach of the control panel. A male colleague stands on a platform at the top of the incline; we are at eye level, ostensibly equals. He chats comfortably with me, a monologue, as I conserve my energy to keep up my stride. I work hard to hide my gasping breath, the stitch in my side, my cramping legs. If I decrease my speed or stumble, I will fall behind. To the people scrutinizing my progress, it will look like I can't "cut it" by comparison.

I talk to a physician-scientist colleague, who also is a gifted ice hockey player. She tells me that ice hockey, more than any of her training, prepared her for a career in medicine and science. To be given a chance on the ice, she needs to demonstrate twice the skill and commitment and endurance and grit as her male teammates. Only then is she granted entry to the "equal" playing field, earning the privilege of having her every move dissected to determine if she can keep up.

The myth of meritocracy tells us that, if a woman simply works hard enough and cares enough about her career, then she will succeed. What no one talks about is how the definition of "success"—what counts as hard work, and how the inputs and outputs are measured and judged—has been historically conceptualized, operationalized, cross-examined, and legitimized by men. The status quo does not account for the hidden labor or systematic disenfranchisement that women disproportionately absorb to stay in the race.

I think about that exhausted first-year fellow, sitting in the front row, eager to learn the secret to "balance." I want to tell her that balance is a holy grail, a sleight of hand. It doesn't exist, at least not in the way that the old guard sells it. Placing "balance" on a pedestal is a red herring: Chasing its siren song distracts us from observing and critiquing the real world behind the mirage.

When a hard-working scientist comes home to have dinner with the kids, we should wonder—and ask one another and ourselves aloud—who planned the meal schedule? Who created ingredient lists, shopped for groceries, and organized the pantry and refrigerator? Who prepared the meal, picked the kids up from school, and shepherded everyone to the kitchen table for family dinner at 6 p.m.?

We need to debunk the premise that anyone can "have it all," particularly on the virtue of hard work alone. When someone achieves "success'" by academia's subjective metrics, we need to recognize and verbalize that their accomplishments invariably occur on the backs of other people's (often hidden) physical labor, emotional support, financial patronage, and experiential sponsorship.

A never-ending mountain of thankless, unglamorous, hard work has to get done, and this labor rarely carries social currency in academia. Unseen work, disproportionately shouldered by women, keeps our institutions afloat, with little, if any, professional benefit to the laborer. In our personal lives, whether stressors include kids or aging parents or home maintenance or any number of other unanticipated challenges, herculean efforts transpiring beneath the surface enable the machinery to function. Without this labor, there would be no grant, no high-impact paper, no promotion, no scientific breakthrough.

After decades of chasing an illusion, I find equipoise in discarding the false dichotomy of "work–life balance." Today, I focus instead on practical, purposeful triage. For me, anchoring my days in triage means that I am mindful and intentional about how, when, and why I choose to invest my energy and time. Sometimes I pour into my clinical work or my research or educational responsibilities; other times, I pour into my children or my friends or activities that bring me joy. Week by week—sometimes day by day, or even hour by hour—I reevaluate how I want to triage my time. There's nothing "balanced" about it, and that's ok.

As I compose my upcoming annual review, I write with an eye for catharsis. I gloss over the line items that affirm my productivity, reputation, and "value" to the institution. Instead, I draft and underline the intangibles—the emotional labor that fills my head, alongside each of the mundane tasks that I juggle to keep my family, community, mentees, staff, colleagues, and institution supported and operational.

I am not naïve. I know that none of this hard work "counts" toward scholarly calculations of my impact or success. But for me, writing it down and talking about it matters. I can imagine a future where we talk openly about the different forms of hard work that we perform in our professional and personal lives. I think it's both visionary and necessary to ask individuals and institutions to recognize and value all types of hard work as the integral pillars upholding academic success. To reach this place, we need to be willing to debunk the archaic fallacy of work-life balance and teach trainees that no one can do it all. We must purposefully grow a culture that incentivizes and legitimizes personal triage computations as a tool for both self-care and self-promotion. Above all, we need to talk openly and vulnerably about the hidden work that drains us and the systems that destabilize or disadvantage us, because we cannot begin to fix what many people do not yet see.

The hard work that each of us triages, day by day, deserves to be recognized and appreciated. For this to happen, those of us who labor beneath the surface need to stop hiding the ripples. It's time to openly make waves.

> Dr. Kaye is a mother, wife, pediatric oncologist, hospice and palliative medicine physician, communication researcher, mentor, and educator. She loves to spend time with her three children, read and write stories, sing, and paint.

A Triumph Over Moral Injury

Joseph R. Betancourt

I couldn't sleep. Our community was being decimated by COVID-19. When patients with limited-English proficiency (LEP) were admitted, not only did they have to fight COVID-19 but they also had to fight to communicate, to understand their caregivers, and to be understood. This was just too much to take amidst all the suffering. We needed to do something.

It was March 2020, just as the COVID-19 pandemic was accelerating in the city of Boston and across the nation. I was asked to help lead Mass General Brigham's effort to ensure equity and community health given my role as Vice President for Equity and Inclusion at Massachusetts General Hospital (MGH). To do this, I assembled a small but amazing team of colleagues and met daily, sometimes twice a day, to craft a plan. As we were getting started, I thought it would be important to create a "multilingual registry" of clinicians, since it was clear we would need to do some major redeployment of staff to meet the impending needs of the pandemic. We put out a call to all those in our workforce who could speak another language in order to find individuals in all necessary settings to help meet the needs of our diverse populations. As a Puerto Rican, native Spanish-speaking primary care doctor who cares for a large Spanish-speaking patient population, I had a unique window into the importance of cultural and linguistic competence.

As was the case across the nation, a large and disproportionate number of MGH inpatients with COVID-19 were Latino/a and Spanish-speaking from our surrounding communities like Chelsea, Revere, and East Boston. Once I became aware of this, I decided to make my rounds on the COVID-19 floors to see how we managed patients with LEP. MGH has a strong and proud interpreter services department that, just a year prior, had delivered over 140,000 interpreter visits via live, video, and telephonic interpretation. However, with the infectious risks of COVID-19, the desire to preserve personal protective equipment, and the need to keep non-frontline workers—including interpreters—out of the hospital, it became clear that we weren't managing those with LEP very well. On the floors, I saw that staff were trying to do their best—using iPhone apps, using family members, and even, in some cases, using children to interpret. This last method was against our ethos and unacceptable in normal times, but the care teams were just trying to do anything they could to manage the crisis in front of them.

During that restless night, I thought about moral injury—when individuals feel they have ignored their conscience or moral compass by failing to prevent actions that go against their values or personal principles. As clinicians, we face moral injury routinely. Due to systemic failures, among a variety of other reasons, we have long recognized the existence—and persistence—of racial and ethnic disparities in health and healthcare. We see that injustices impact all patients but disproportionately impact vulnerable patients. Research has demonstrated that when compared to the majority population, minority populations not only die at higher rates from some of our nation's largest killers such as diabetes, cardiovascular disease, and cancer, but also receive a lower quality of care for a variety of condition within the healthcare system even when they have the same level of insurance, or health status. There have been many times in my career where I have felt heartbreak as the system in which I practice medicine falls short for patients of diverse backgrounds, and I was afraid I would see it happen again for these Spanish-speaking patients with COVID-19.

The following morning, I racked my brain as to how we could do a better job caring for our Spanish-speaking patients with COVID-19. By this point, they comprised 40% of our COVID-19 inpatient census. At a minimum, I could start rounding with the surge teams so I could help bridge the language gaps.

As I played with this idea, it slowly started to hit me: Since we had already put together a multilingual registry, what if we culled the list for native Spanish-speaking physicians to assess their willingness to help? Many of my colleagues had been sidelined because we had shut down various services, such as surgery and pediatrics, and they were either being redeployed or had been redeployed already. Why not take advantage of their bilingual capacity and redeploy them to assist with communicating with Spanish-speaking patients? The "Spanish Language Care Group"—or SLCG—was born.

We spent the entire week working on building and operationalizing the SLCG. An incredible 51 native Spanish-speaking doctors, from 15 clinical disciplines, and representing 15 Latin-American countries, answered the call. They ranged from a renowned professor of surgery to a junior pediatrics faculty member to an orthopedic resident—and many others. The physicians were ready and able to serve their community in any way possible.

We constructed a work plan that included the need for seven doctors during the day from 7 a.m. to 7 p.m., four doctors at night from 7 p.m. to 7 a.m., and a doctor in the emergency department 24 hours a day—all working shoulder to shoulder with the medical teams, on all floors. Our introductory Zoom meeting explained the process, answered questions, and brought us together as the SLCG. To say it was inspiring was an understatement. I have never been prouder in my career to stand with my Spanish-speaking peers, willing to put themselves at risk with all the unknowns of COVID-19 at the time, to make sure that at every bedside of a Spanish-speaking patient with COVID-19 there would be a Spanish-speaking doctor, working with the medical team to ensure cultural and linguistic competence for every encounter.

Within two weeks, the medical teams knew how to access the SLCG, and we were fully integrated into the clinical care of Spanish-speaking patients. We participated in discussions when patients were admitted, when patients were being discharged, when patients were consented for clinical trials, when patients were visited on during daily rounds, and, in the hardest moments, when patients had conversations about serious illness and the end of life. We spoke to family members, near and far, including all across Latin America, letting them know how their admitted loved ones were doing, and, in worst cases, letting them know their loved ones were about to die or had already died.

Medical teams began to depend on us and expected us to be there. They really understood our contributions to patient care and the importance of diversity in healthcare. Our colleagues were blown away to see how clinicians who brought clinical, cultural, and linguistic competence to the daily encounters fundamentally improved the communication, quality, efficiency, and effectiveness of clinical care. Day by day, we earned their trust, respect, and praise.

The patients also depended on us and expected us to be there. When we walked into a Spanish-speaking patient's room, through all the masks, face shields, goggles, and gowns, they simply heard, "Buenos dias! Como se siente hoy?" (Good morning! How are you feeling today?) The sense of relief, knowing that they would be understood, and they could communicate, brought invaluable and immeasurable joy that was visible in their faces. The SLCG had succeeded in its mission to improve the quality of team-based care of patients with COVID-19 and LEP—in the most compassionate, caring, and culturally competent patient experience possible.

Finally, the first surge of the pandemic began to wane. Our COVID-19 inpatient numbers dropped significantly, as did the demand for the SLCG. Over the previous six weeks, we had provided a service to MGH, to Boston Hope (a major field hospital in Boston), and later even staffed the telephone lines to help patients obtain outpatient monoclonal antibody infusions. We filmed over 15 videos in Spanish on all topics related to COVID-19 that were distributed to the community. We did Facebook videos and interviews, served as trusted messengers, and brought key information to our community in a language they could understand.

The six weeks of that first surge had created an incredible win–win–win: Patients loved being cared by Spanish-speaking doctors; the medical teams loved having us by their side; and we absolutely loved being able to come together as a community, to serve our community. Through the crucible of the first surge, the SLCG had forged an incredible bond, built on love for our community, respect for each other, and an incredible sense of commitment and dedication to honor what brought us to where we were in our profession, at that moment in time and in history. We could all proudly say that when duty called, we answered the call. Hopefully we saved some lives and made many lives better along the way.

In the end, the SLCG remains the single most important and most special effort I have ever been a part of, and this memory will undoubtedly last a lifetime. While moral injury can feel like a losing battle and be emotionally devastating to the physician, there are occasional wins when creativity, dedication, and teamwork come together to develop an action plan. Through the SLCG, courage, diversity, and cultural competence triumphed over moral injury.

> Dr. Betancourt is the president of the Commonwealth Fund, an Associate Professor of Medicine at Harvard Medical School, and a board-certified internist, providing primary care to a large Spanish-speaking and minority patient panel. He has devoted his career to improving the quality and value of healthcare for diverse populations.

Forging Trust

Andrea Reilly

"Don't you trust me?"

As soon as the words left my lips, I could not believe I had spoken them aloud. I perceived a shift in the room, felt my own body stiffen. The patient and her mom greeted me with stares. Even if I had thought it—the words should not have slipped out. The tone of the visit changed. I had let them know my frustration. In the adolescent's eyes—that rarely met mine—was a question: *"Whose side are you on? Because if you're against my mom, I'm against you."* So much for winning over my patient.

One year earlier, at our first visit, I was drawn in by the troubling history. The school turmoil had started more than two years prior. The mother spoke rapidly. Her daughter had initially been bullied by a group of girls on the bus. She became withdrawn. The parents started driving her to school. Once, the bold middle-school tormentors even followed alongside the car, yelling chants. She stopped going to school altogether. She began to wear her bangs long, obscuring her face. She became thinner and thinner. The daughter attended therapy—sometimes. The mother arranged for her to be home-schooled. They no longer went out together as a family. The daughter refused to eat in restaurants and became very anxious leaving the house. She rarely left her room.

I wanted to help. We spent nearly an hour together at that first meeting.

At subsequent appointments, I spoke directly to the silent daughter, seeking to connect. There was a deep sadness in her gaze. We explored her interests in music—she especially liked percussion. I listened to the nervous mother. She was ardent to navigate her daughter through a turbulent adolescence but was entangled in her own self-doubt. She, too, had lived a childhood of upheaval. In our shared moments, I laid the groundwork for collaboration. Time, I hoped, would lead to trust.

Fast forward to this visit. The day had been a busy one. By the third patient of the day, I was already running behind. Still, I spent time with the patient and her mom. The exam room phone rang. It was the medical assistant: "Your next two patients are waiting." The appointment was wrapping up—or so I thought. We had spent the better part of an hour discussing progress in some areas—no change in others. I listed the age-appropriate vaccines she was due for and was about to leave the room.

That's when her mom took a step back and said, "Oh I have to think about that." I reiterated what I had said at previous visits about safety and tried to allay concerns. The parent continued to decline, telling me, "Well, I want to do my own research." I was flustered and annoyed at this point. I had already spent more than the allotted time in the room, trying my best to provide understanding and good care, and then this?

I looked at her and asked, "Don't you trust me?" As soon as the words left my lips, I knew I had said too much. I recommended the Centers for Disease Control and Prevention website, suggested a close interval follow-up, and left the room.

I had another six hours of patient appointments—but that interaction gnawed at me.

Three days later, I was notified that the parent had called and told our practice manager it was "not a good fit." They would be finding a new pediatrician.

Perhaps I should have sensed it. I had been very gentle in the beginning—listening, commiserating about the prior treatment mishaps and uncompassionate caregivers—but then I saw the entire story unfolding before me. This teen would be turning 18 soon, and there were conditions I should address before they got even worse. I had fallen into the trap of thinking I would be the savior.

Compassion and empathy are crucial for physicians, but becoming emotionally invested so that you feel let down if the patient or parent disagrees with you is too much.

As I had gotten to know the patient and her mother better, I learned how their life had plummeted downward, and I yearned to make a difference. I became bolder in my comments. I outlined the importance of working in concert with a therapist, mental health team, and a nutrition team. I encouraged the teen to relieve panic attacks by exercising and getting an app for her phone. I offered frequent follow-up appointments.

Caring for a teenager is always a challenge—as a parent, teacher, and doctor. As a med-peds physician, I am attuned to this awkward transition phase since I care for young and older patients as well. But throw in a pandemic coupled with fragile self-esteem, and coping mechanisms of caregiver and patient are overwhelmed. The role I strived for in this case was as advocate, health advisor, and healer. I saw myself as a broker, trying to work on a doctor–adolescent–family partnership. As I tried to ally with the parent, however, we diverged.

I am still trying to improve this coalition. When parent and pediatrician are aligned, all goes smoothly. However, my role supporting a parent also includes highlighting ongoing health risks to a child, even if it seems impolite. I pointed out to the parent that her daughter's refusal to leave the house due to paralyzing anxiety was worth trying a medication. I did not say this at visit #1 or even #2; but by visit #3, I spoke up. I saw the desperate eyes before me. And I also remembered my older patients who struggle as adults: a 24-year-old patient who has been in and out of the ED continuously due to emotional dysregulation; a 47-year-old adult who has not left the house in years. Perhaps they each could be coping if a careful treatment plan had been instituted when they were children. I wanted to intervene.

Until now, I had prided myself on working with all-comers. Since I began medical practice, my patients have included families on alternate vaccine schedules. It was a change from the usual pediatric care guidelines, but I reasoned some vaccines are better than none; and later is better than never. But I have also seen more and more young adults with chronic medical problems that could have been mitigated in childhood. At that moment I blurted out, "Don't you trust me?" I was unable to keep a straight face and pretend it did not matter if a child with a BMI of 17 eats one meal a day. Part of my frustration was my shock at the parent's not partnering with my ideas. I did not see them as *my* ideas. I saw them as the general pediatric recommendations for a child this age with these illnesses. But in the parent's eyes I was no longer a teammate, I was a foe.

So here I struggle. I am mad at myself for not expressing my point of view in a more persuasive and kind way. I fell short of my intention, to provide guidance while building a trusting, open relationship. While I cannot ignore the dangerous patterns I see before me, I can still work on the way I address them. How do I walk this line?

The approach I took was too blunt. As much as the apprehensive teen had improved in comfort level with me in the last year, I miscalculated the fragility of the parent. And for this I am sorry. I got it wrong.

My exasperation bled through and I lost sight of the goal: to build one teenager's confidence, make her feel valued, and create a desire to overcome her challenges. I left out the parent for a moment, and the fragile scaffold of trust we were constructing fell apart. Perhaps I should have pulled the mother aside to spend more time talking one-on-one about what had worked so far and what hadn't. I was so focused on reaching the teen that I missed reacting to the fear and concern in her mother's eyes. She knew things were not going well. She knew this child was disconnected, different from her other children, isolated from classmates. Each failed treatment attempt reflected on her. Of course, she wanted to do the best she could. She had so little control over the process of an anxious mind. But vaccines—now there she could say yes or no. And if there was any chance something harmful was going to enter her child's body, she was about to prevent it.

I wish we had had another visit, time for another conversation. I am awash in a strange mix of heartbreak and righteous despair. I am grateful this is not the end of the story. The teen found another doctor closer to home and is making slow progress.

Doctoring is a humbling profession. Some days I don't get it right. I struggle with dueling obligations: a duty to prevent harm and a duty to recognize one's autonomy—even if that may put one at harm. Such is the dignity of risk. There is an elegance and beauty in laying the groundwork by explaining pathophysiology, reviewing treatment options, and then stepping back to allow individual (or parental) decision-making. But there are many gray areas. I wish to speak and convey the message of prevention clearly, kindly, but with ardor. I'll call this gentle force. But for all of this, my day-to-day is frequently about getting through my lab results, patient notes, and trying to stay on time. I blurted out my self-doubt when I asked,

"Don't you trust me?" I was really saying, "Please trust me." At my core, I believe we are here not to judge but to take care of one another.

> Dr. Reilly enjoys dancing, skiing, and cooking with her family. Favorite moments include hiking in the White Mountains with her dog Lia. Professionally, her joys come from teaching new parents how to enjoy parenthood and watching adolescents come into their own. Her work with survivors of trauma and human trafficking has brought her is touch with the beautiful resilience of the human spirit.

Being Fired

Michael Jellinek

Ethical, productive, academic doctors almost never get fired, and doctors in senior administrative positions, although more vulnerable, are rarely "replaced."

But this happened to me. For those who face a similar circumstance, the experience can feel like a trauma. It is a substantial personal loss, because we put tremendous pressure on ourselves and invest heavily in creating our professional identities when that identity is gone, we are no longer whole. I was fired and faced that loss, as well as the emotional and practical consequences.

I started as the Chief of Child Psychiatry at Massachusetts General Hospital (MGH) and an Instructor in Psychiatry and in Pediatrics at Harvard Medical School (HMS). I was 30 years old and had trained in pediatrics at Montefiore in New York City, general psychiatry at MGH, and child psychiatry at Boston Children's. I could not imagine working at a better place than MGH and was thrilled to be offered a low-paying job that I was not ready for! My career blossomed. Over the next ten years, I built a nationally recognized department and competitive residency program while publishing in peer-reviewed journals. I was promoted to Assistant and then Associate Professor, and to Associate Chief of Psychiatry for Clinical Services. Throughout this period, I had the help of excellent colleagues, generous mentors, and wonderful Chairs, Dr. Tom Hackett and then Dr. Ned Cassem.

The next phase of my career started in 1990, when I was one of three physicians given administrative titles at MGH. I became Vice President (VP) of Ambulatory Services with oversight for 800,000 visits annually, a process improvement team, and a member of the hospital executive leadership team. In 1996, I was promoted to Senior VP of Hospital Operations with responsibility for approximately 20 department heads with 3000 employees. In 1997, I was promoted to Senior VP for Hospital Administration, with added responsibilities for space management, long-term master planning, radiology, pathology, pharmacy, and compliance with approximately 5000 employees. Academically, I continued to publish and was promoted to Professor of Psychiatry and of Pediatrics.

In early 2000, I was asked to lead a turnaround of Newton Wellesley Hospital, a community-hospital affiliate of MGH that had lost $54 million dollars over 48 months. With the essential help of a superb team over a 12-year period, the hospital became one of the best in the state, with a four-fold growth in clinical revenue, margin of 4%, and the highest patient satisfaction scores in the system. In 2012, I was asked to take on a system-level role as the Chief Clinical Officer, with oversight on quality, and leading a $1.2-billion-dollar five-year implementation of EPIC, a new and complex electronic medical record system. In October 2014, I received my annual review and was told I was doing well, on-time and on-budget with EPIC, given an "A" and 100% of my bonus.

Thirty days later, I was fired! They asked me to stay on for 6 weeks to help the new Chief Clinical Officer transition into my position.

Within minutes, my 38-year career in the system, including nine administrative and three academic promotions, ended. I was out of my large, walnut-paneled office overlooking the Charles River: no work, no secretary, no reserved parking space, and no long-term fringe benefits.

The first feeling was a massive sense of loss. I had been a part of this health system since age 27 and had many deep, long-term relationships that I had enjoyed immensely and routinely, and I now felt those core friendships were at risk. At the age of 65, with retirement savings and a generous severance agreement, my concerns were not financial. However, the culture, the people, the routines, the locations, the safety of what was familiar, and what I was devoted to were gone. When I came home and told my wife, she thought I was joking. My bonus check had just cleared into our account.

Why was I fired? I suspect that cultural tensions within the system were not sufficiently addressed (by me or anyone else in leadership), and the implementation of EPIC across two major academic medical centers in the same system, compounded by the fear of conflict, kept the concerns below the surface. I decided not to agree to the usual announcement about my leaving and refused to accept an email memo explaining "that I wanted to spend more time with my family" or "that I decided to retire." I instead asked the announcement of my leaving to state that I was either "fired" or "replaced" by the CEO, which would allow me to be honest with all of my many professional and personal relationships. With corporate reluctance, the announcement was drafted my way. I negotiated to keep my hospital appointment so I could continue to use my email account, teach the child psychiatric residents, and participate in a research group.

The day after I was fired, I went to a senior mentor who gave me three recommendations:

1. Put the past behind you. Endless or obsessive thinking about this complex political situation will not be enlightening or helpful.
2. Be good to yourself for the next year in whatever way that matters to you. Recover from this event.
3. Start networking today if you want to continue working. Look around and consider every option—academic, administration, consulting, and so on. Do not wait to network during the six-week transition.

Not everyone has a relatively easy adjustment to being fired, and that is because of a critical framework that put my reaction into perspective. Five years earlier in 2009, I experienced a much more profound, tragic, and overwhelming loss: My second son, Abe, had a drug-related death.

Abe was a brilliant 24-year-old who suffered from intractable depression and anxiety. His IQ, especially in the verbal subtest, was near genius (he read chapter books at age 4), and his depression on testing was among the most profound an experienced, expert psychologist had ever seen. Abe was so depressed at age 14 that he almost needed to be hospitalized. Using grit, he completed a demanding high-school program and, despite being a humorous and sarcastic critic, won the faculty award at graduation for best representative of the school's values. His college thesis was a discussion of whether artificial intelligence would blur the line between machine and human consciousness. He wrote this in 2005. As you can tell, I was very impressed by him and loved him very much.

We, especially my wife, did everything within our power and made every sacrifice at every age to help Abe survive and enjoy life. He received flexible, empathic care from his mother from infancy, as a breath-holding toddler, as a child who read late into the night, and as a sensitive, depressed teenager. His brothers and sister looked past, as best they could, his moods and anxiety, to his inner caring and dazzling intelligence.

After his death, we learned his drug use was not recreational, but an attempt at relief and a replacement for the prescribed psychiatric medications that had no impact on his anxiety and depression other than uncomfortable side effects. Hindsight tortures us. If only we had known about the drugs and forced Abe into a rehabilitation program against his will… but we balanced those doubts with an understanding of how forcing Abe to do anything would have crushed his soul and an awareness of how much he suffered every day.

Abe's death made every member of an empathic family more empathic. It put every other loss and disappointment into perspective, including the potential loss of my professional identity and the fear I had of losing 38 years of relationships.

After Abe's death, the family functions well, and we find joy in our children and grandchildren. We remain grateful for what Abe gave all of us. But recovering from that loss? Never. Recovering from being fired? Absolutely.

Three months after being "replaced," I started as an Executive VP in a new system with oversight of community hospitals, clinical departments, and population health. I would have liked to be in my old job seeing my former colleagues more often, but working in a new system gave me a fresh perspective and new experiences. I retired from working in hospital systems in 2017 after another merger. At age 68, I chose the option to return to MGH, to teach, see patients, write, and have a practice coaching and consulting with CEOs of about a dozen companies of various sizes and industries, rather than immerse myself in another new system.

Losses are a stressful, inevitable part of life, when aspirations in sports, academics, family, and jobs do not come true. How one copes with loss is instructive and often consistent from loss to loss. While I have experienced the well-known stages of grief—denial, anger, bargaining, depression, and acceptance—everyone has their own reactions to loss. The stages vary in length and intensity, and our personal reactions can include harsh self-criticism, poor self-care, and even substance use. If you are fired, do not get selected for a job, or have a major loss in your personal or professional life, think about my mentor's advice. "Putting the past behind me" prevented me from dwelling or perseverating. "Treating myself well" implicitly told me I am a deserving person who should not be too self-critical, who should accept losses as largely beyond my control. "Starting to network immediately" helped me initiate planning, focus on what I had control over, and resulted in very positive feedback from others wanting to help and employ me. For my job loss and especially the death of Abe, talking to my family and close friends and repeatedly grieving together were essential as there is no substitute for empathy from those close to you.

> Dr. Jellinek continues to see patients, consult, and teach. He and his wife have three wonderful adult children (two criminal defense lawyers and a school resource officer) and six granddaughters. He enjoys his hobbies of woodworking, blacksmithing, and the never-ending struggle to lower his golf handicap (currently 14). Dr. Jellinek acknowledges the contributions and editing of this essay by Abe's siblings, Isaiah, Hannah, and especially David.

Caregiving

3

Kathy May Tran, Marc S. Weinberg, Susan Hata,
Laya Jalilian-Khave, Michael Natter,
Vinayak Venkataraman, Emmett A. Kistler,
LaShyra T. Nolen, and Sandeep Jauhar

K. M. Tran (✉)
General Internal Medicine, Department of Medicine, Massachusetts General Hospital, Boston, MA, USA

Department of Medicine, Harvard Medical School, Boston, MA, USA
e-mail: kathy.tran@mgh.harvard.edu

M. S. Weinberg
Memory Disorders, Department of Neurology, Massachusetts General Hospital, Boston, MA, USA

Department of Psychiatry, Massachusetts General Hospital, Boston, MA, USA

Department of Psychiatry, Harvard Medical School, Boston, MA, USA

S. Hata
General Internal Medicine, Department of Medicine, Massachusetts General Hospital, Boston, MA, USA

Medicine-Pediatrics Residency Program, Massachusetts General Hospital, Boston, MA, USA

Department of Pediatrics, Massachusetts General Hospital, Boston, MA, USA

Department of Pediatrics, Harvard Medical School, Boston, MA, USA

L. Jalilian-Khave
Department of Psychiatry, Yale School of Medicine, New Haven, CT, USA

M. Natter
Endocrinology, Diabetes, and Metabolism, Department of Medicine, New York University Langone Medical Center, New York, NY, USA

Department of Medicine, New York University Grossman School of Medicine, New York, NY, USA

V. Venkataraman
Sarcoma Center, Department of Medical Oncology, Dana-Farber Cancer Institute, Boston, MA, USA

Department of Medicine, Brigham and Women's Hospital, Boston, MA, USA

Department of Medicine, Harvard Medical School, Boston, MA, USA

© The Author(s), under exclusive license to Springer Nature Switzerland AG 2024
M. A. Goldstein, K. M. Tran (eds.), *Becoming a Better Physician*,
https://doi.org/10.1007/978-3-031-69413-4_3

E. A. Kistler
Department of Medicine, Harvard Medical School, Boston, MA, USA

Critical Care, Department of Medicine, Mount Auburn Hospital, Cambridge, MA, USA

L. T. Nolen
Harvard Medical School, Boston, MA, USA

S. Jauhar
Cardiology, Department of Medicine, Northwell Health, New Hyde Park, NY, USA

Commentary: Deep Breath

Marc S. Weinberg
I'm flicking the mouse wheel
Scrolling through a ribcage into dense white clouds
And scattering labs on my notes sheet like tea leaves
When I hear an alarm.
In psychiatry, alarms mean fire
But we're not in psychiatry
And the workroom comes alive
Everyone grabbing their gear, and emptying
Into the hallway.
"Your faceshield—you're not wearing your faceshield!"
Her hands reach up and poke through the empty space where her shield would have been.
Her eyes widen and she backs against a wall.
I'm third in line.
An intern steps down and another climbs up
And presses hard against the young Black man's ribcage
Expelling virus from his lungs
In a great big plume.
They parachute down across the room
All the way to the woman against the wall—
But she left, and the door is closing back on us
Vacuum restored.
It's my turn to press, and I press hard
Looking straight down at him.
Another plume of air shoots out past his front teeth
Hitting my shield.
I breathe out through my nose,
Like in swimming.
Warm air leaks out past my mask
On the right side
Towards my eye.

I press again and watch his mouth
No tube. No mask. Jaw open.
This time they shoot straight towards the breach in my mask
I breathe out forcefully from my nose
And hold my breath.
His heart restarts, and the room empties.
I follow his bed out of the unit
And head towards the bathroom,
Close the door, unmask, and pull my face close to the mirror.
Indentations of the mask remain on my cheeks. Except in that one spot
On the right side
Towards my eye.
Ma'am, your son is fighting hard. He had a … he's moved to the …
We're breathing for him now.
He's in good hands. Of course. You're welcome.
He died.
Home, I strip down by the entryway to my apartment
Scrubs and socks and shirt shoved into a white trash bag
I pull the plastic strings and compress it down.
A plume of air whooshes past the drawstrings
Out into the foyer.
I hold my breath,
And watch all the tiny parachutes
Drift slowly to the ground.

> Dr. Weinberg is a physician-scientist researching novel treatments for psychiatric illness and memory disorders. He lives in Stoneham, Massachusetts, with his wife and two baby girls.

Befriending Our Edges

Susan Hata

Just after the New Year in 2021, I walked into the medical ICU with three lattes and a jar of lentil soup. I had arrived at a lull in Saturday afternoon rounds, and I had never seen the ICU so silent before. Every room was full, but every door was closed. Not a family member was in sight in the hallways. This was the dark winter of the COVID-19 pandemic. As the residents turned from their computers to accept the refreshments, a nurse touched one of the interns on the shoulder to say that a patient had just died and needed to be pronounced dead. The intern stiffened and paused and then stood up. The senior resident quickly said, "I'll go. You stay for a minute." She walked across the unit and began arraying herself in a yellow gown, gloves, and an N95 mask outside the patient's room. Her movements were reverent and calm.

One of the other residents said, "Every patient here has COVID. This happens," gesturing to the senior resident, "multiple times every day." The intern stayed silent while the rest of us chatted, her eyes focusing on the door of the patient's room where the senior resident had disappeared. She turned to me and distantly thanked me for the coffee. I thanked her for working over the holiday. "This is the first time I haven't been home for Christmas," was all that she said. Not wanting to keep them from their work, I walked out of the unit feeling that coffee and soup and thanks were inadequate balms for the suffering I had just witnessed.

The work of caring for patients and their families brings us to the edges of ourselves again and again. We brush up against the limits of our knowledge, our physical energy, our clinical reasoning, and our emotional resources. When I was a resident, it happened in the early hours of the morning at the bedside of a sick patient, or when my pager awakened me, or when my inadequacy was exposed on rounds. As a primary care doctor now, something as simple as a call from radiology can mean a conversation that changes a patient's life forever, and an unkind word from another can unmask depths of weariness I didn't know I carried. In those moments, the work that I love is asking something important of me, and I'm not sure I have a worthy answer. Suddenly the edge of my abilities feels dangerously close.

For a long time, those moments felt so distressing that I tried to avoid and protect myself from them. I worked harder, double-checked my clinical reasoning, and went to great lengths to communicate carefully and build relational connections. While all of that effort to be perfect made me a better doctor in some ways, it also wore me down and it didn't make me feel safer. The thought of sustaining that degree of stress for another 30 years until retirement felt impossible. Yet the thought of leaving medicine made me feel even more lost. I had trouble imagining a way to stay in the job I loved without being destroyed by it. One day, in my journal, I wrote, "I just want to feel at home in my work." Coming home. It was an image that filled me with relief and hope.

At that time, my kids were small and full of energy and also brought me frequently to the limits of my capacity. To stay sane, my children and I went out exploring nature at every opportunity. We walked Crane Beach, collecting seashells, looking for piping plovers in spring and snowy owls in winter. We explored the Arboretum near our house, collecting pinecones and seedpods, and learned to recognize the coming of spring by the flowering of the rhododendrons, then the mountain laurels, then the lilacs. My favorite path led through the woods, under the shelter of huge old trees. Standing there, knowing the trees around me had thrived through years of sun, wind, and snow, I felt safe.

What if we can befriend our edges, not as cliffs over which we might fall, but as the tips of branches? Branches are alive, and when they grow, they *push their edges back*. Like a spreading oak tree, as our edges grow, we open, we become more spacious, we become a refuge for others, we become stronger at the center.

To plant ourselves at home in the world requires cultivation. It requires care and attention and patience—all habits of tending, of being tender, with ourselves and one another.

For me, learning these new habits means unlearning some old ones.

As I sit with patients or go through my lab results, I practice holding uncertainty with gentleness rather than guardedness.

When I know I've made a mistake and feel disappointed in myself, I let compassion come alongside shame and remember that repairs are possible.

As I drive home, I notice the concerns that I still carry with me from the day, and instead of resolving to check the charts again that night, I choose to transition to time with my family. Being at home in my work is easier when I allow myself to be at home at home.

Slowly, these practices are working on me, expanding my capacity to love and engage, rooting me deeper in solid ground.

It's been two and a half years since that COVID-19 winter day in the ICU with the residents. Sometimes, I think I understand what this pandemic has given to us and taken from us and, other times, I'm sure I don't. But I keep coming back to the memories of that senior resident stepping in to spare her intern another deathbed pronouncement, of that intern quietly naming her first Christmas far from home—pictures of tender care. My children are old enough that now they lead the way on our hikes through the woods, and they point out to me when the oak trees are dropping the acorns that will nourish the squirrels through the winter. The decades between me and retirement are starting to feel more like a friendly invitation than a chore. Who knows what lies ahead—what life will ask of us? Perhaps when we feel afraid, when the ICU is full, when the world changes and we're at the limit, tenderness can push the edges back, and can be our path home.

> Dr. Hata enjoys providing primary care to children and adults, teaching residents, and supporting physicians in the joys and challenges of their professional lives. She creates spaces for physicians to reflect on their experiences through support groups, Balint groups, writing groups, and retreats. Dr. Hata is pursuing a Masters in Fine Arts in Creative Nonfiction from Pacific University.

The Art of Listening: Beyond Languages and Borders

Laya Jalilian-Khave

A woman in her thirties shows up at a refugee clinic because she is having trouble becoming pregnant. She is a refugee from a remote village in Afghanistan, and she arrived in the United States a few weeks ago. I am a medical doctor and postdoctoral trainee from Iran, shadowing the clinic team to gain experience. I had arrived in the United States a few months ago.

She has been trying to get pregnant for years. Taliban had taken over Afghanistan, and she and her husband had to flee the country. I can only guess how much pressure she must have carried with her through the years without any clue as to why she could not have a child and lacked the health resources to find out why.

She has been diagnosed with Turner's syndrome, a random genetic disorder that led to a missing sex chromosome. It has some distinctive characteristics and symptoms, including infertility, but sometimes it is not evident by someone's appearance. This is the first time she will hear such news. I cannot even guess how much pressure she is destined to carry now, knowing how her life has turned over since leaving everything behind to create a safe future for her family.

We walk into the room with the attending physician and the medical intern. She talks in Urdu, a sibling to my mother language, Farsi, and I can understand almost half of it. It's the first time I've heard it from a patient since I immigrated, and I find it calming to listen to her tone. She looks surprised and delighted when I faintly say "Salaam"—the Farsi and Urdu word for hello. The intern tries to simplify the genetic condition as much as he can, and I recognize a similar struggle in his face that I recall from my own face years ago.

"All of us are born with chromosomes. One pair is related to our sex, and most women have two X chromosomes. You only have one. This explains the period irregularities you mentioned. We should first monitor you for heart, kidney, and metabolic problems. Then we will walk you through the next steps."

He pauses after every sentence for the interpreter to translate, looking at the patient with patience and empathy. She just nods uncomfortably.

"Do you have any questions I can help with?"

She asks shyly, "So I got this disease from my husband?"

The intern gets frustrated and repeats his explanation again.

She can't look at him, ashamed and feeling out of context. She is on the verge of tears, "So how did I get this from my husband? He wants a child now. What was the heart problem again?"

The frustration escalates in the room. I can't hold myself back anymore and whisper to the attending, "She doesn't get the chromosome part. She probably has no biology or anatomy background. All she hears is the word sex, and that probably directly points to sexual interaction in her cultural background."

They explain to her differently this time, and she comprehends some parts or at least acts like it. She says thank you, how grateful she is, waiting impatiently to leave the room, with an anxious heart that she was told might not deal well with anxiety. She waits to meet her husband at the door. She probably does not have the words to describe the new and dramatic shift in her life.

Language and cultural barriers in healthcare systems have been discussed as threatening patient care and patient–caregiver relationships. The two, closely intertwined and inseparable, are among the healthcare systems leading causes of disinformation and relationship asymmetry. Was it the lack of words that built up the wall between her and the rest of the room or the cultural gap?

The interpreter was using her words but not the way she knew them. The doctors were telling her strange things about her body, but not the way she knew herself. It was about the words, and it was not.

When the language is not shared, we see our differences more boldly. The easiest concepts are lost in translation, and if our words are different, then so are our contexts, cultures, upbringings, and lives. However, we might also see our similarities more boldly. The hardest concepts rise beyond the words. We know we want the shared value of life, care, and love, once we look at each other in the eyes.

I look at the intern's uncomfortable face, and my thoughts return to the months before I came here.

Back in Iran, after graduating from medical school, I moved to a remote hospital in a village at the border of Iran and Afghanistan to do my service. You think you know how to swim while you are close to the beach. You take another step further into the sea, and suddenly, the ground disappears from under your feet, and you realize you don't know how to swim well enough to deal with the sea.

It was my first independent medical experience. With an anxious heart, I had pulled all the strength in me to bury the nervousness, the naivety, and the fact that I did not know how to swim in that depth with a professional-looking face. It was a different dialect and accent, and when those two were not the barriers, our two dissociated universes stood out. One could say that my patients and I had never lived in the same country. To them, I repeated myself over and over for days, until I realized I was talking too fast, and I was using words that were not getting through. I asked about the nature of the symptoms over and over again, until I realized there were not so many words there to describe the pain or even understand the pain.

"It feels like a kind of pain in the chest." I pull up my list of cardiac chest pain symptoms in my head. "It's crushing, like hopelessness, but crushing, you know…? Because I don't know, I just want some medication for tonight," he continues. This time, I am the one out of context, and I have no choice but to knit myself within their threads and lines, learn to swim in the deep side off the beach and between wave after wave of poverty, war, and pain that I had just watched from the comfort of the beach.

In medical school, we are trained to learn the patient's history by using a questionnaire, framing human suffering within a few words—our own words—and putting it in the chief complaint. As vital and necessary as these skills are, we tend to forget that pain cannot be framed within this questionnaire or any questionnaire, and the same goes for life. Regardless of the depth of the gap between words, cultures, and worlds, the human sitting in front of us will frame and mold our questionnaire, any questionnaire.

The language and cultural differences in the healthcare system are rapidly growing on both ends. The number of immigrants grew to 281 million in 2020. That's 3.6% of the world's people, which is undoubtedly reflected in patient care systems. While we should be conscious of these barriers and how to address them, we can simultaneously see these barriers as a chance to remind ourselves more than ever that we, the medical team and the patients, are fighting for the same value: life. That is a reason to drive us to try harder to place ourselves in our patient's shoes, to listen carefully and to discover their words and worlds, as well as our brief time together might allow. This practice is about the words, as in a different language or words as in the same language, but in different contexts. Listening is about words, and it is not. It is much more than the words and much more than the worlds words create. It is about fighting for life.

> Dr. Jalilian-Khave is a general physician, a postdoctoral fellow in the Department of Psychiatry at Yale School of Medicine, and a Public Voices Fellow of the OpEd Project.

One to One

Michael Natter

There is a distinctive scent I have come to associate with the inpatient ward of a hospital. It is an amalgam of sterile cleaning agents, body odor, and stale bed linens. I've smelled it while lying on the rickety cot in the resident call room, rounding in the ICU at 4 a.m., and making my way down the hallways of the medicine wards. There is no inherent positive or negative quality to this smell, but it is plainly characteristic. It is what my olfactory bulbs, after years of inpatient indentured servitude, have come to label as uniquely "hospital." My mind has other fragrant associations, too, like the unmistakable scent of oil paints and charcoal dust from my undergraduate days spent in the art studio. Those were decidedly pleasant smells—inspiring, even. That connection of smell, memory, and emotion is visceral to me.

A year out of training, that inpatient odor had faded away into the recesses of my limbic system, tucked away with the other sensory experiences of arduous medical training that I was not sad to catalog away. That is, until it crept back into my nasal passages—only this time while I was standing in the elevator heading to a locked inpatient psychiatric ward of the hospital where I had trained. A visitor's tag had replaced my resident badge, and that familiar odor was now mixed with the scent of my mother's perfume.

She was almost unrecognizable. Mental illness had taken over, and she became depressed, angry, anxious, tortured—a prisoner of her own mind. She would act out in illogical and frightening ways—outbursts, both physical and emotional. Dark, deeply hurtful words flew from her mouth, each stinging me like lashings from a whip. This was the fifth inpatient hospitalization in a string of many since her mind became poisoned nearly five months before. In between hospitalizations, I would be awoken by phone calls from emergency physicians informing me of another new and bizarre presentation. I would recite to the attending on the other end of the line a memorized history of my mother's course while still partially asleep. The exhausting journey in navigating her treatment was taking a toll on her, on my family, and on me. No one seemed to know what was happening, what to do, or who could help.

Before medical school, when I was an art student, I held the false belief that medicine existed in the binary: black and white. Diagnostic tests would solidify pathology. Treatment modalities would cleanly eradicate the etiology. The prognosis would be clear and definitive. Instead, what I found was that medicine is much more like my familiar art world than I would have thought. It exists in the gray—perhaps no field more so than psychiatry. There are no X-rays to identify the fracture to be set, and no A1c to assess the need for higher insulin dosing. In my training, I had come to realize this uncertainty, and having a protective cloak around me in the form of a white coat allowed me to come to terms with this nebulous ambivalence. Once I found myself in the role of advocating for my mother's health, with no protective layer to distance me, the ambivalent gray had become intolerable. It swallowed me whole. It was tortuous. Sleep was elusive. Appetite was gone. I was waking up at 5 a.m. to help my mother get to inpatient treatments, running to my own clinic, and then biking back to her hospital bedside, pedaling through snow, rain, cold. I was a doctor—a healer—and this was my mother. I needed to fix her but I was entirely helpless to do so.

As a doctor, I have seen a lot. Training in a New York City public hospital, I've shouldered unimaginable loss, strife, and ethical challenges. Yet, even when the world crumbled around me in the spring of 2020, as I found myself dead center in the eye of the storm caring for patients in the COVID-19 ICU, nothing could have prepared me for this experience at the bedside of my own mom. It was hard to step out of my clinical persona. My identity as a healer meant that I should be able to save my mother. I should be able to solve this medical puzzle. But medicine does not work that way. There is no complete certainty in what we do, and no guarantee of exact diagnosis, treatment, or cure. I've spent considerable time counseling patients and their families on just that. And yet, despite this insider knowledge and my deep understanding, on the other side of that doctor-patient relationship, my other identity as a son grappled with accepting that uncertainty. As my mother unraveled, I did, too. My knowledge, skill, and experience as a physician were useless, and I was powerless. No matter how hard I tried to gain control, I had none and I eventually needed to give up trying to grasp for any.

While I ceded control as a physician, I never gave it up as a son. In doing nothing—or at least feeling as though I was doing "nothing" as a physician—I had an epiphany. I didn't have to be a doctor—only a son. I couldn't do anything medically to make my mom better. But as a son, I could do a lot. I could be there. I could support her in her illness. I could hope for healing. And that's all I could do. I couldn't cure her. I couldn't determine the trajectory of her mental illness. But I could be present.

There was liberation in this recognition of what I could and could not do. The anger I was harboring had eased into a sadness but also a hope. I reached a point of peace. I stopped intellectualizing and finally took the advice I had given my patients so many times before. The gray was all around me, but I was accepting it instead of fighting it. Reminiscent of my days covered in charcoal, late nights in the art studio staring at my art, knowing there was no right or wrong, there was no answer, no definitive answer, just the ability of choosing how to deal with the reality of what was around me.

As the months continued, my mom's mental health gradually and miraculously improved. Her mind calmed, and the pain of her tortured thoughts faded. However, the new perspective of my epiphany did not. Like the other realizations of medical training, it took feeling broken to make myself whole again. That dichotomy of being a physician and a son was an inflection point that drove home that unfortunate truth that despite how much we want all the data, all the information, we will never have full answers. It is the nature of what we do as physicians and it is the nature of who we are as human beings. Engaging with that uncertainty and accepting it can be not only extremely painful but also liberating. Life can be full of despair and periods of suffering. It is natural to question our place in these moments. I believe one of the many jobs of a physician, like an artist, is not to succumb to this despair but to find an anecdote to these dark points. Often, that anecdote is not necessarily in intravenous fluids or a surgical procedure; it can be simpler than that.

My mother no longer has the scent of the hospital on her, but the memory of that scent traumatized and scarred me. Yet, this scar acts as a reminder of the other side of the doctor–patient relationship—what patients and loved ones go through. I now approach my patients and their families with a deeper understanding of the frustrating interface between patient and sickness and our convoluted health systems: acknowledging the gray of medical practice within them, recognizing the difficulties of uncertainty and the feelings of helplessness, sharing in the frustration with them and the human condition that is inherent to us all as we go through our own illness and that of our loved ones.

> Dr. Natter identifies as an artist, humanist, and physician. He is passionate about infusing his background in studio art into his medical practice and education. Diagnosed with type 1 diabetes in childhood, Dr. Natter understands the medical experience from both sides of the exam table and aims to make medicine more humane, artistic, and empathetic.

Young Hearts Dying

Vinayak Venkataraman

My second year of residency:
- I see him lying in bed, tangled in wires and tubes. His thin beard covers a youthful 20-something-year-old face, his head rests in a puddle of unkept hair. His chest, covered each morning with stethoscopes, showcases unfinished tattoos.
- He's in the cardiac ICU (CCU) because of his mangled, failing heart. He requires powerful medicines to keep his heart pumping.
- I am in the CCU as a rotating junior medical resident.
- He's a difficult patient. I see him be mean and lash out, not follow the rules, push others away.
- But I also see a kid who grew up healthy and became fatally ill, whose hopes of independence were thrown into disarray.
- I listen as he tells me his tortured life. He tells me he was mistreated growing up, spending those days in and out of juvie. "Those were the best years of my life. How screwed up is that?" He tells me he's homeless and jobless due to his heart. He has limited support beyond his girlfriend whom he loves.
- I feel a strange desire to get to know him better each day. I see the judgments that have smothered him his whole life and try to wipe a bit off each day.

His heart will continue to worsen. We try but cannot turn off the powerful medicines that sustain him. His only hope is a heart transplant. It's unlikely he will leave the CCU without receiving at least a ventricular assist device (VAD).

The cardiology, cardiothoracic surgery, and intensive care attendings had met the day before and decided neither VAD nor transplantation would be offered at our hospital.

I walk into his room.

He turns to me. "What up, bro doc?"

I love that name. We've become close. We're both from Upstate New York and love music and football "You like the Bills, man?" I had asked. "Hell no, bro, they're so bad! Though I guess the Giants suck too."

I sit on the edge of bed, level with his eyes. We bump fists, then shake hands, then lock knuckles, and hold. I place my left hand on his right shoulder.

He doesn't wait. He asks, "So, doc, am I getting a VAD or what?"

I pause. He reads my face.

"It's bullshit!" he yells. "I've sacrificed so much! I gave up everything I like for this. How's it my fault I'm homeless? I couldn't work with this stupid heart. You'd use weed too if you were in my place."

He shakes his head. "I could have just died happy, livin' my life, doing whatever I wanted, but now I'm stuck here with nothing to look forward to."

He takes a deep breath. We continue to grip hands.

I know he's heard this news before, but I feel supreme guilt as its latest communicator. I told someone who allowed me into his life that we're not going to do what is necessary to save his life.

"I knew this would happen, man, and I know what I want," he says, "I want y'all to get me on the meds I need."

I fear he might leave *against medical advice*, as he's done before.

"And I want y'all to get me back home."

He continues, calmly, "I wanna die in peace, comfortably, in my dad's house."

I remain silent. So does he.

Minutes, which feel like hours, pass as we both look down, breathing heavy breaths. He releases his hand and grabs his phone.

He calls his dad, "I'm not getting a VAD, Dad. I'm coming home… to die. I'll see you soon." And abruptly hangs up.

He calls and tells his girlfriend, adding, "I told you they'd never give me one, why did I listen to you?"

He turns toward me. "I appreciate you, bro. I'm not trying to be rude or nothin'. But I need some space."

I nod. Before leaving, I look him in the eyes and say, "I wish you didn't have to tell me what you just did. But now we know, and we'll do everything we can to make it happen."

He briefly smiles, then nods, dejected.

We bump fists, clasp hands, and slowly let go.

I walk out of his room, engulfed in devastation.

I'm outraged for the hand he was dealt. Outraged for all his life has lacked in love and support. I wish I could prescribe him that.

I'm outraged and sad that he is going to die. That there's nothing a young trainee like me can do.

I'm shaking. My senior gives me a hug and sends me outside. I escape the unit's overwhelming orchestra of alarms. My idealistic rage is tempered as I pass by rooms of patients with VADs whose bodies are being consumed by strokes and infections. I'm reminded of how much can go wrong when medicine pushes the boundaries of life.

I walk outside to a quiet Sunday evening, bury my head in my hands, and cry.

A few minutes later, I lift my head, dry my eyes, and head back for the remaining 12 hours of my 24-hour shift.

I check in on him as the CCU nurses check in on me.

He smiles and invites me to make myself comfortable. I sit on the end of his bed and grasp his hands again. I ask, "How are you doing, man?"

He replies, "I'm better."

We sit together as he begins to grieve.

He's been thinking about his death for quite some time. He approaches it with a mix of eloquence and humor.

He tells me, "I was a *bad* person," before meeting his girlfriend and being diagnosed with heart disease. "I know I got my flaws," he says, "but I try to be a better person today than I was yesterday."

He tells me how much he loves his girlfriend's young daughter. "She's been acting out more since I've been gone."

"I wanted *so bad* to walk her down the aisle," he adds. He tells me the song he had picked out for their first dance. "That shit's my jam!"

"I guess that ain't happenin'," he says. "It is what it is. That's how life sometimes goes, I guess."

We talk about his dad's house. I ask, "Is that a special place?"

He replies, "Yeah, man, I love it. It's out in nature and so peaceful." He pulls out his phone and shows me pictures of a large house surrounded by forest. He shows me his dad's retro car collection. He's excited to drive them when he gets back home. He shows me pictures of his family, his dogs, and himself as a kid.

He tells me about the dreams he had that he'll never accomplish (he wants me to know he had dreams).

I promise to do everything I can to fulfill his final dream—to get back home one last time.

His mornings are filled with unrelenting depression.

He tells me, "I'm a good person," and asks, "Why am I the one who has to die? Why do others deserve a heart but not me?"

I have no words. I retreat back to gripping his hand and shoulder and telling him how much it all sucks and how sorry I am.

I know he's been told his entire life that he's worthless, and each day, I do everything I can to make him feel worthy.

Initially, I'm scared he won't be going home. He's so sick, requiring so much support. I know how devastating that would be—to die in the CCU.

But he slowly turns a corner. His young body mends. Potent medications start coming down, then off. A week later, he's finally on just one through his veins. It's a powerful one, rarely used outside a CCU. But one that patients like him can take at home to keep them going until they die.

I'm on call on July 4. We play desktop ping-pong in the afternoon. He tells me he wants to watch the fireworks outside with me.

I can't go down initially, but I am able to escape for the last ten minutes. I walk outside and see him across the street in his wheelchair. I come up from behind and tap his shoulder.

He turns and smiles. "Bro! I'm so happy you made it."

"Wouldn't miss it for anything, man."

We look back toward the effervescent sky.

I ask, "What's the best fireworks you've ever seen, bud?"

"Oh man," he replies without thinking. "The best was back in Albany. I was five or six or something like that. I remember being so scared, all those loud noises and shit. But it was the most amazing thing I'd ever seen."

"All that fire and fury."

"Hell yeah."

"How've these ones been?"

He pauses, then smiles.

"Beautiful."

For a few minutes, I see him light up like the sky, smiling the whole time. He feels completely free and unleashed, joy overcoming his underlying sadness. The fresh air and camaraderie rejuvenate his spirits (and mine).

We watch together as colored flames thunder up from the Charles River, into the white-dotted sky, explode into red, orange, and purple stars, and rain down over us both.

A few days later, he is discharged and makes it back to his father's home. He reconnects with his family and community, and they rally to fulfill his "last three wishes": a motorbike parade, a wedding, and a pig-roast reception. He marries his girlfriend and becomes a husband and stepfather in a well-attended ceremony filmed by the local news. A few days later, he passes away, comfortably, at peace, amid loved ones, with dignity and beauty.

Six years later, I have finished my medical training. As I start my life as a medical oncology attending, I think back to this patient. I remember the details of this experience so vividly; however, I am now able to maintain distance from its newness, rawness, and brutality, and appreciate the lessons I have since learned.

I have found fulfillment in supporting the physical, emotional, and social health of young adults as they face critical illnesses during a critical period of their lives. I appreciate my care of young adults differently. I'm no longer age-matched as I was in training. I forge connections now by simply asking them, with compassion and curiosity, to share with me their goals, their dreams, their fears, their lives. And I've also learned I need to balance my prior "vigor, intensity, and love" with self-preservation and emotional balance.

I still care for my patients as if they were my family, but I do so knowing they are not my family (and they don't want or expect me to be). I avoid becoming so closed and wrapped up for these lines to feel blurred.

As an attending now, I can see this patient through the lens of the attendings who supervised me. Their decisions were hard and gray, without clear winners or right answers. "Easy decisions," like offering a VAD to a young dying patient, can cause undue harm, such as debilitating stroke due to nonadherence.

It is often harder and takes more time to say "no" to life-sustaining treatment, even when it may be what is best. I feel this way now when I share that chemotherapy will do more harm than good and hospice may be the best approach.

I am proud of myself as the resident who stood up for and supported a young patient I grew to care deeply for. I am honored he invited me into his life during those weeks, and I remain immensely proud of our team's efforts in honoring his dying wishes. I am also proud to be an attending now, who strives every day to provide the very best care to all of my patients, but who also works hard to establish balance, boundaries, and expectations in my practice.

> Dr. Venkataraman is a medical oncologist with expertise in caring for patients with bone and soft tissue sarcomas. He is also an internist and pediatrician with expertise in supporting the physical, emotional, and socioeconomic needs of adolescent and young adults (AYAs, age 15–39) facing cancer. He is interested in leveraging novel technologies and artificial intelligence to improve cancer care, research, and outcomes. He is also a published essayist with passion for creative and reflective writing in medicine.

Tell Me More

Emmett A. Kistler

As a medical student, I led a project called "Tell Me More." Other medical students and I asked hospitalized patients about what was important to them and their favorite memories. I heard stories about cooking attempts gone laughably awry, parents who worked two jobs to help get their children through school, and legendary dance moves passed down from father to son. Many patients wept as they spoke. We cried, too.

While the patients shared their stories, we wrote the highlights on bright yellow dry-erase posters and, as if they were trophies, hung them in prominent locations in the patients' rooms. When nurses or doctors entered the room, I watched as their facial expressions softened and their body language relaxed as they took in the "Tell Me More" posters. Sometimes, more conversation about national heritage or pets ensued. Sometimes, it didn't. We left the posters up for as long as we were allowed.

As I prepared to start residency, "Tell Me More" was humanism in medicine come to life. It was an opportunity to connect with patients as individuals rather than compilations of medical problems. It was also a space for patients to reflect and define what was important to them in the midst of an illness. Those bright yellow posters also served as a wake-up call to the providers who were too busy or forgetful to ask these questions themselves. Afraid of losing the humanistic spirit, I vowed not to become one of those physicians.

As a resident physician just a few months later, this vow was tested early and often. Compared to medical school, the hours in the day felt scarce as I learned how to juggle patient care, career interests, and my own well-being. Most of my time was dedicated to understanding pathophysiology, testing indications, and principles of management—an unending compendium of knowledge that loomed over the intern year. Despite program-wide attempts to emphasize compassionate care through coaching efforts, reflection sessions, and, yes, even the same "Tell Me More" posters displayed in our patients' rooms, the humanistic aspect of care I once championed drifted quietly out of focus.

This drift was never more apparent than during an inpatient medicine rotation in my second year of residency. For a month in the late spring, I led a service with high acuity and turnover. Each day felt like a sprint from start to finish. As if being timed, I limited my interactions with patients to several questions, a cursory exam, and a hollow "see you later" as I ushered my team to the next task. I could feel my muscles tense up if the patient interview wandered off-topic, at which point my mind oscillated between a daunting to-do list and the optimal way to end the discussion.

About a week into the rotation, I met Bobby Bird. He was a 65-year-old man with Down syndrome, and he was admitted after an aspiration event precipitated severe hypoxemia requiring high-flow nasal cannula. Bobby looked tired as we entered his room and greeted his family. Glancing regularly at his sister Debbie, he offered only a handful of words during our interview. After examining him, we hashed out a plan for antibiotics, dietary restrictions, and moved on.

Several days passed and Bobby's oxygen requirement continued to teeter on 100%. Reviewing his medical history more closely, the initial impression that this admission was due to an isolated pneumonitis evolved into a more concerning picture of chronic dysphagia, progressively worsening lung function, and a potentially terminal aspiration event. "Discuss goals of care" became a daily task.

Each day, Bobby's family made an hours-long trek to sit at his side and listen to our updates, which grew progressively grimmer. After days of referencing worsening lab data and imaging, we held a family meeting and recommended against intubation and other invasive end-of-life measures. His family, however, remained optimistic and felt strongly that he receive every measure possible. I pushed on, bringing more objective data to the family to make our case that such interventions would do more harm than good. We cycled through the same conversations, and our interactions with Bobby's family became fixated on the end of his life as he lay in bed, still watching us quietly.

After more than a week into his admission, our attending mentioned that Bobby had starred in a television show. Seeking solace from discharge summaries that evening, I found myself doubled over in laughter and tears clicking through video after video of Bobby Bird.

Bobby was a reporter, a musician, and an actor. He co-starred in an MTV comedy/documentary series called "How's Your News?" that aired in the 2000s. He and other members of Camp Jabberwocky, a sleepaway camp for people with disabilities, road-tripped around the country and asked the titular question to celebrities, politicians, and passersby on the street. Bobby unabashedly approached everyone from alligator farmers to U.S. Secretaries to get to know them—to ask his version of "Tell Me More"—with pure, unrivaled enthusiasm. In one scene, he brings comedian Sarah Silverman to joyful tears. In the next, he pumps his fist excitedly after snagging a few moments with singer Will.i.am on the red carpet.

Before rounds the next day, I asked everyone to pause what they were doing, and I pulled up YouTube. The air in our work room felt lighter and time seemed to slow as we sat with big grins on our faces watching Bobby zoom around the screen. After several videos, we took a moment to recognize not only our collective surprise and delight from learning about Bobby Bird but also remorse for not doing so earlier. We shared our findings with Debbie and the rest of his family later that day, and our learning continued. We heard about Bobby's favorite foods, his antics at camp, and—nonchalantly mixed in with other stories—his conversation with John McCain. Bobby smiled knowingly as his sister spoke.

Debbie also opened up about other aspects of Bobby's life. She told us about how trusting and loving he was, and how people had tried to take advantage of him in the past. Debbie shared how protective the family had become of Bobby, and how that defensive attitude now applied to medical decisions. She expressed that Bobby deserved every opportunity available during life, as well as at its end.

Previously fixated on his oxygen saturation and chest X-rays, my attention was now drawn to the sheer contrast between the quiet man in the corner room and the vibrant reporter touring the country. I wasn't the only one to notice this difference; revisiting prior facets of Bobby's life brought the magnitude of his present illness into focus for our team as well as for his family. We continued our conversations with Debbie in earnest, focusing as much on Bobby's life as we did on the prospect of death. Learning more about Bobby and understanding his background did not make these conversations any less difficult, but the daily checkbox and the associated outlook were no longer part of the routine.

Over the ensuing days, Bobby's oxygen saturation drifted downward despite maximal support. A host of friends and family came to visit, including folks from Camp Jabberwocky. Bobby was eventually transitioned to comfort-focused care in discussion with his family, and he passed peacefully in his sleep one morning toward the end of my month on service. Debbie and I hugged as she arrived to take Bobby home.

During my pulmonary and critical care fellowship training throughout the COVID-19 pandemic, Bobby Bird came to mind frequently. Rounding in the ICU, I recalled fondly the many conversations I had with Bobby and his family in person—an unknown luxury at the time—as hospital visitor policies were adapted to meet infectious risks. Weighed down in N95s, face shields, and gowns, I found myself stealing extra moments in patients' rooms, reading through the "Tell Me More" posters so I could report on the information to my team alongside the physical exam and ventilator data.

With so many patients intubated and removed from their loved ones, learning our patients' stories required more effort than ever at a time when our capacity to make those efforts felt frustratingly limited. Even with so many obstacles in place, though, missing the human side of patient care—to only know a patient as the 65-year-old man with an aspiration event and severe hypoxemia—felt like a disservice to our patients and to our role as clinicians.

Years after being introduced to the phrase, "Tell Me More" still embodies humanism in medicine. Reflecting on the vow I made as a medical student and the circumstances of the pandemic, however, I've tried to take a more forgiving approach when there isn't time or a way to ask. Rather than a wake-up call, I think of "Tell Me More" as a gentle reminder to revisit the humanistic side of patient care when the day affords me a moment.

And I remain grateful to Bobby Bird, who pointed out that this phrase is as important to the patient and their family as it is to me as their physician.

> Dr. Kistler is a pulmonary and critical care physician in Cambridge, Massachusetts, who focuses on patient safety and quality improvement. When not in the ICU, he enjoys running around town with Moose, his Labrador Retriever.
>
> Dr. Kistler acknowledges and thanks Bobby's family, especially his sister Debbie, for all their care of Bobby, for sharing his story with us, and for giving permission to write about him.

Superheroes Need Healing Too

LaShyra T. Nolen

"I'm doing fine. Don't worry."

Her words normally cut through the air with power, but this time was different. This time her words were fragile. They floated. I listened, trying to be their safe landing pad, but I felt helpless.

She was sick, we were at the peak of a pandemic, and I was in medical school more than 3000 miles away. That year I was completing my clinical rotations at a safety-net hospital in Cambridge, Massachusetts as a second-year medical student. Our patients were among the sickest in the Greater Boston area, and many of them had COVID-19. I spent my days wearing N95 masks and yellow gowns, hoping the next patient wouldn't be someone I loved. But it felt inevitable.

The fragile words on the other side of the phone were those of my mom—the most important person in my life. Born and raised in Compton, California, she raised me as a single parent and was the first in our family to go to college, obtaining both her bachelor's and master's degrees. Her brilliance was the foundation of my curiosity for learning, and her resilience inspired me to accomplish any dream I set my mind to. Because of her, I became the first Black woman to become student council president in the history of Harvard Medical School. This year I will become the first physician in our family. It will be our greatest accomplishment to hold together.

My mom has always been my "why" and, in many ways, my superhero, but it seemed like this time she was the one in need of saving. At first, I convinced myself to believe her pleas that she was "okay," but with each phone call she sounded a bit weaker. The pauses between her coughs got shorter and shorter. I was worried. The latest variant of COVID-19, alpha, was plastered over the news and was deemed by scientists to be more severe than the previous variants. The new vaccines were recently approved by the Food and Drug Administration but, unfortunately, they still were not available to the general public. I was concerned the dreaded virus might have caught her.

Despite the knot in the pit of my stomach, I told my mom she should take a COVID-19 test. With luck, she was able to find an open appointment at a local testing center, and we held our breath waiting for the results to return. On a Wednesday afternoon, I opened a message with a screenshot that read: "Positive for SARS-CoV-2." My heart dropped to the floor. Trying to remain calm, I explained to her the meaning of the results and that she should call our family doctor immediately. While my mom was young without significant comorbidities, I was still concerned, not only because I loved her but also because she was a Black woman.

As a medical student researcher with a budding career in studying the ways racism impacts health outcomes, I was especially aware of the consequences of her reality. COVID-19 was ravaging America's Black communities. Black folks were more likely to contract COVID-19 and to die from it because of lack of access to testing and treatment—both testaments to how the illness exacerbated the sociopolitical inequities that existed before. Health organizations and the media were swept away with the narrative that Black patients were "vaccine-hesitant" and did not want the vaccine, but there was no conversation about vaccine access. For these reasons I founded "We Got Us," an organization to bring health information and vaccine access to Black communities in Boston.

Before the pandemic, medical racism was well-documented in several clinical domains. Studies demonstrated the biases that physicians have toward Black patients, incorrectly characterizing them as having an increased pain tolerance and dubious symptom presentation. Similarly, studies about the inability of pulse oximeters to detect hypoxia due to the darker skin of Black patients emerged as a major concern during the pandemic, as this was a standard indicator for disease severity. I wondered how the harrowing reality of medical racism and health disparities would impact my mom's care if she ended up in the hospital.

As I listened to my mom's words floating through the air, scared and nervous about her new diagnosis, these data swirled through my mind, along with questions that tugged at my heart: *Will they make her another statistic? Will they believe her? Will they treat her with dignity? Will they provide her with the best care? Will they treat her like she was their own mother?*

I was in a virtual afternoon clinic when I found out the results. As I treated patients and made up care plans, the knot in my stomach never left and my heart remained on the floor. I couldn't stop thinking about her. While I trusted my future medical colleagues, I knew that no one could advocate for her the way I could. I had to be her advocate. I had to be her medical student. I had to be home.

Even though I was in the middle of a clinical rotation during the busiest time of medical school, the most important patient of my life needed me. I spoke to my clerkship director, and they immediately worked out a plan for me to continue my clinical training virtually and return home to care for my mother. I boarded a plane that evening with my N95 masks and stethoscope, along with the medical knowledge I gleaned over my 15 months in medical school.

As soon as I arrived home, I worked with our family physician to create an outpatient care plan and a list of contingency options if her condition worsened. I spent my days doing hourly vital checks and pulse oximeter reads, while preparing medications and meals. My mom's fragile words were no longer coming across the phone but through her mask. While it was difficult to see my superhero wounded, holding my stethoscope to the chest of the woman I admire the most helped me see her humanity in a way I never had before. She needed a safe space to take off her cape, a safe space to be human.

Today my mom continues to save the world, but now I give her powerful words space to be fragile and her resilient spirit space for rest. The experience of caring for her taught me that even superheroes need saving. In healing those heroes that inspire us most, we may discover there is a superhero inside of us who deserves healing too.

> Ms. Nolen is a physician activist, leader, and writer with a deep commitment to serving and advocating for marginalized communities. She is the founder of "We Got Us," a Boston-based grassroots nonprofit committed to the promotion of healing and antiracism. Her writing centers on themes of Black healing, justice, and reparation. She will be completing her internal medicine residency at Brigham and Women's Hospital.

My Father Didn't Want to Live if He Had Dementia—But Then He Had It

Sandeep Jauhar

Two years ago, when my father was dying of dementia, my siblings and I faced a terrible dilemma: whose wishes for his medical treatment were we to honor? Those of my father back when he was a healthy, highly functioning geneticist? Or those of the simpler weakened man my father had become?

It was a predicament that has led me to rethink my views on advance directives for end-of-life care.

At the time, my father's health had been in decline for several months. His appetite had been steadily decreasing, he'd been losing weight, and he often had to wear a diaper because he couldn't always make it to the bathroom in time. Now, he had taken a rapid downturn over the course of a week, and he had stopped eating and conversing.

Thinking he might be dehydrated, my older brother and I, both doctors, started to give him fluids through an IV at home. It didn't help. We were faced with the awful choice of whether to remove the IV and withdraw medical care.

Some years back, in 2004, my father had written a letter to my brother saying that if he or my mother were to get "very sick," neither would want extraordinary measures taken to keep them alive. "We want to live only if we have a meaningful life," he wrote. In keeping with my father's directive, formulated when he was "of sound mind," my brother said we should stop the IV fluids and let my father die peacefully.

I had misgivings. It was true that life in a state of dementia would not have seemed meaningful to my father in 2004. The scientist in him would not have wanted to live without an intellectual existence.

But, despite his weakened state, my father didn't seem unhappy. Over the course of his illness, he'd never expressed a sincere wish to die. What was meaningful to my father in 2004 was very different from what had become meaningful to him in the past few months, when watching TV, spending time with his caregiver and children, and even just eating a spoonful of ice cream had clearly given him genuine pleasure.

It was possible to view those pleasures as simple, childlike, somehow beneath my father. But wasn't this man before me also my father? Why not continue the IV fluids, I thought, and maybe try giving him some antibiotics?

This is a conundrum that in one form or another many families are facing. At the hospital system where I work, almost half of the 600 or so ethics consultations performed last year dealt with various disagreements over advance directives. "It is a daily occurrence," Renee McLeod-Sordjan, the head of our bioethics service, told me.

The sort of problem my siblings and I faced will only increase as the population ages. The number of Americans estimated to have Alzheimer's or related forms of dementia is more than six million today and is projected to double in about 25 years. Many older Americans will have advance directives like my father's. And in many cases those directives will seem to contradict their current desires.

Courts have generally ruled that an advance directive should be prioritized as an expression of the will of a person when he is presumably independent and rational and has the time and the presence of mind to reflect on what he wants. However, isn't that also a kind of bias that risks lowering the moral standing of the patient in later years? A person's current wishes, even if formed in a state of cognitive impairment, must count for something. As a son, how do you withhold life-saving treatment from your demented father who, through gestures and utterances, seemingly expresses a desire to live?

My brother often said that my father was living a life of "plus-minus," by which he meant that it basically added up to zero. In my darkest moments, I believed this too. But perhaps we were suffering over our father's condition more than he was. His world had shrunk, but so had his desires, his perspective, and his expectations of what constituted a worthwhile existence. The man who'd craved recognition and respect more than anything else no longer seemed to care about those fickle rewards.

To my brother, our father was no longer the person he once was. To me, he was still the same person, just a changed one.

In the end, after much debate, my brother, in conjunction with a hospice nurse, made the final call to honor my father's advance directive, which is the goal of palliative care. We stopped the IV fluids and did not start antibiotics. Our father died at home a few days later.

I continue to struggle with the question of what caregivers should do in this situation. Perhaps a family dispute such as ours might be avoided if an advance directive were to state explicitly that the contrary wishes of a "future self" should not be heeded, though this still would not resolve the ethical dilemma.

Though courts may disagree, I no longer believe that advance directives should strictly be followed in every situation. They are often vaguely worded and may poorly predict future attitudes and feelings. To me, it seems that a contemporaneous desire to live, even in a person with dementia, must be taken seriously, despite what that person might have previously written. We recognize that minds evolve and people change in every sphere of human life.

Families and caregivers should weigh both past and present wishes in deciding what is in an incapacitated patient's best interests. This would be best accomplished by a surrogate in tune with the patient's wishes and how he has evolved—in most cases, a loved one chosen by the patient in advance. Ideally, social norms will one day reflect this.

As I learned on the journey through my father's illness, contentment with life can be compatible with cognitive dysfunction—along with the prerogative to change one's mind about the care one wants at life's end.

My journey also reminded me of how important it is for physicians to remain involved with their patients near the end of their lives. In fact, the end of life may be when familiar physicians are needed the most. I still remember how much I appreciated my father's internist staying in touch with us during those fraught days. I aspire to do that now with my terminally ill heart failure patients.

In our medical system, physicians are taught to seek cures. We often become frustrated when diseases enter a terminal phase, reminding us of our impotence in the face of death. I used to be one of those physicians. I would step back when my patients entered hospice care, thinking their care could be managed exclusively by palliative specialists. But my experience navigating through the end of my father's life reminded me that trusted doctors are needed at every stage of the life cycle.

Dr. Jauhar is the author of *My Father's Brain*, named a Best Book of 2023 by *The New Yorker*. He is a cardiologist at Northwell Health and writes frequently for the opinion page of *The New York Times*. The original version of this essay by Dr. Jauhar was first published in *The New York Times*.

Physician as Patient

4

Mark Allan Goldstein, Paula K. Rauch, Carrie Cunningham, Emily M. Herzberg, Rana L. A. Awdish, Emily Silverman, Peter Grinspoon, Giuseppina Romano-Clarke, David V. Diamond, and Evonne Kaplan-Liss

---

M. A. Goldstein (✉)
Adolescent and Young Adult Medicine, Department of Pediatrics, Massachusetts General Hospital, Boston, MA, USA

Department of Pediatrics, Harvard Medical School, Boston, MA, USA
e-mail: mgoldstein@mgh.harvard.edu

P. K. Rauch
Child Psychiatry Service, Department of Psychiatry, Massachusetts General Hospital, Boston, MA, USA

Department of Psychiatry, Harvard Medical School, Boston, MA, USA

C. Cunningham
Endocrine Surgery Program, Department of Surgery, Massachusetts General Hospital, Boston, MA, USA

Department of Surgery, Harvard Medical School, Boston, MA, USA

E. M. Herzberg · G. Romano-Clarke
Department of Pediatrics, Harvard Medical School, Boston, MA, USA

Newborn Services, Department of Pediatrics, Massachusetts General Hospital, Boston, MA, USA

R. L. A. Awdish
Pulmonary Hypertension Program, Pulmonary and Critical Care, Department of Medicine, Henry Ford Health, Detroit, MI, USA

Department of Medicine, Michigan State College of Human Medicine, East Lansing, MI, USA

Department of Medicine, Wayne State University School of Medicine, Detroit, MI, USA

E. Silverman
Department of Medicine, University of California San Francisco, San Francisco, CA, USA

P. Grinspoon
General Internal Medicine, Department of Medicine, Massachusetts General Hospital, Boston, MA, USA

Department of Medicine, Harvard Medical School, Boston, MA, USA

© The Author(s), under exclusive license to Springer Nature Switzerland AG 2024
M. A. Goldstein, K. M. Tran (eds.), *Becoming a Better Physician*,
https://doi.org/10.1007/978-3-031-69413-4_4

D. V. Diamond
Medical Department, Massachusetts Institute of Technology, Cambridge, MA, USA

E. Kaplan-Liss
Center for Compassionate Communication, T. Denny Sanford Institute for Empathy and Compassion, University of California San Diego, San Diego, CA, USA

Department of Pediatrics, University of California San Diego Health, San Diego, CA, USA

Commentary: There Is No "Us" and "Them" in the Doctor–Patient Relationship

Paula K. Rauch

Facing one's own medical illness as a physician is an unwelcome but powerful teacher. Every such experience I have faced highlights the importance of collaborating with patients to build a healing doctor patient relationship. One that respects and integrates their lived experience.

My experience with a neurologic migraine during pregnancy that mimicked a stroke was a powerful early career teacher. The transient field cut, aphasia, and right-sided numbness differed markedly from my medical school textbook knowledge. There was no black triangle like the quadrantanopia in the book. The experience of no words and an inability to read and comprehend felt mysterious. The ordinary objects I looked at without words seemed to have heightened beauty and color when I could not locate their names in my blank brain. My arm was not without sensation; it felt like it was enormous and bloated with an odd numbness. Only when my ability to speak returned along with the numbness did I feel the fear that persisted after the experience. The anxiety about whether it would recur, and if so, when and where, is unforgettable. It was a masterclass in the difference between knowledge learned from a book and what is learned through lived experience.

So much of my medical school and residency experience focused appropriately on diagnoses and treatments. There is so much to learn. I deeply admired the brilliant diagnosticians that I was fortunate to learn from, yet most of my 40-plus years of clinical practice has focused not on making the dazzling diagnosis, but on helping patients live well with the challenges of medical illnesses. I have come to recognize this as the core of being a physician.

Mortality is easy to measure; morbidity is more elusive and personal. It is easy for a physician to underestimate the impact of a patient's symptoms and, without a clear treatment, to offer the patient to withdraw. Symptoms matter in quality of life. I have had my life teachers with a couple of bouts of crippling back spasm, a kidney stone, and the dramatically misnamed condition of benign paroxysmal vertigo. Vertigo is anything but benign!

On the other side of the doctor–patient relationship, I deeply appreciate the physicians who stay connected even when they do not have a fully effective treatment to offer me, the ones who listen with curiosity, respect, and compassion to my lived experience. I have weathered my symptoms better thanks to their continued engagement. I am reminded that my patients, too, deserve a physician who remains engaged without the unconscious or explicit expectation that my recommendations must be deemed effective, or I will withdraw. Connection, engagement, caring, and the simple act of timely response to a patient's calls, especially when there is not something to do, are powerful tools of healers.

In the end, there is no "us and them" in the doctor–patient relationship only "us and us." I am grateful for my excellent medical education, mentoring, and colleagues' support—each contributing immeasurably to my ability to be a better physician. The knowledge of diagnoses and treatments is essential, and our patients deserve a current and knowledgeable physician. I am also grateful for the lessons learned from the lived experience of being a patient. The latter has played a key role in growing my compassion and my humility, both essential to this privileged calling of being a physician. As a senior physician, I anticipate a future of more lessons learned from being a patient.

> Dr. Rauch is a child and adolescent psychiatrist whose clinical work focuses on the impact on children of medical illness in the family. She recently stepped down from directing the cancer center parenting program that she founded and continues to teach, supervise, and mentor. She enjoys consultation work outside the hospital including a long-time collaboration with PBS children's programming, long walks, and time with her husband, adult children, and grandchildren.

There Is No Crying in Surgery

Carrie Cunningham

Two thousand people sit completely silent. No scrolling, no chatter. There is palpable anticipation. Expectation turns to anxiety the longer it takes me to start speaking.

I look down at my word-for-word speech. I repeatedly read the first word, a simple "yes." I think to myself, "Just say the first word." Then I say this aloud. I start to cry, and the audience begins to clap in encouragement. *There is no crying in surgery.* I make a joke and get a lot more laughter than it deserved. A bit of release for everyone.

I am trying to do something that is against every ingrained behavior I have—against the narrative that I have so meticulously crafted for my entire life. I am about to share my mental health story with a room full of surgeons.

I am not a religious person, but I do acknowledge the sense that some things are meant to be. If there was ever anything I was supposed to do on this planet, it is to share this story, at this moment in time, to this group of people. I have never been surer of anything in my life.

I finally begin. I dedicate the address to my friend (and fellow surgeon), Tina Barkley, who died by suicide in 2012. Her sister, Jill, is there in the front row. More tears. I read the entire first page choked up, taking frequent breaks to (sloppily) blow my nose.

Over the course of the next 40 or so minutes, I outline the course of my mental health crisis and treatment course over the past year. I divulge that I am a person with lifelong depression and recent diagnoses of post-traumatic stress disorder (PTSD) and substance use disorder. I explain that despite all of my professional success (I am giving the speech as a Presidential address of the Association of Academic Surgery), I am not immune to human suffering. I am not special. I describe in detail how I felt and feel, about shame, fear, and hopelessness.

I talk about the epidemic of suicide in healthcare workers—doctors and nurses have twice the suicide rate of the general population, and the results of an anonymous survey of those seated in the room. One in ten respondents of the survey admitted to suicidal ideation within the past 2 weeks. I repeat, "One in ten of you," and pause to let it sink in. The majority reported knowing a colleague who has attempted or died by suicide. A tenth acknowledged substance use disorders and only a quarter had ever sought treatment for their own mental health. I say out loud what we all think—that we fear we will lose our jobs and our reputations if we seek help. I say what I fear from giving this speech:

> "There will be jobs that I am not offered, there will be doubts as to my abilities, there will be people who see me as weak, emotional, and damaged."

I then try to get to the heart of it. I implore everyone to put health first, take care of one another, and don't believe it when someone says they are fine if you know that they aren't. I talk about identity, self-compassion, and the ugly side of perfectionism, as well as the importance of discerning profession from identity. And their health is more important than the ability to practice medicine.

…suffering isn't a competition.

…there aren't two teams, caregivers versus caretakers.

…the universal need for authentic connection to yourself and others.

I try to motivate those in the audience to change, to think differently, to get involved in making things better, to hold space with others who are struggling, to allow themselves to grieve their patient losses.

I feel the weight of those in the crowd suffering in silence themselves. They are nameless and faceless given the glaring lights. I am scared that I will not say the right thing, and that I will have the opposite of my intended impact. I state plainly that their feelings are valid, and that depression doesn't equal weakness. Depression says nothing about competence as a physician. Recovery is a brutal but critical process of deep inquiry, brutal honesty, and self-compassion.

I feel relief and pride as I conclude and receive a standing ovation. At the time—as a person still in the raw stage of early recovery—I think, "Ironic to be given a standing for being in rehab." I now know that they were applauding courage and providing support for the others struggling around them. I will never know if, how, or whom I helped or hurt. I was compelled to try. Something had to change. It was the right thing to do.

Since that day, many have reached out to me privately applauding my vulnerability and sharing deeply personal stories, which is the foundation of successful recovery. People in recovery like mantras: "connection is protection." Thousands of people have viewed the YouTube recording of my speech, and millions read the *Guardian* article. This was not about me, though, it is about igniting change. That someone else felt the things they felt. The timing was right. It resonated.

My story is not unique. I had the privilege of job and financial security. I had built a practice and reputation. Our trainees and students do not have these resources to fall back on. Just as their education and competency is our responsibility, it is our responsibility to provide a safe and supportive environment to grow as human beings and to afford them the right to *be* a human being.

So be brave with me, please. Whether that means seeking help for yourself, reaching out to a struggling colleague, or advocating for infrastructure changes. If nothing else, learn about the resources at your institution, what state physician health programs offer, and try to use appropriate nonjudgmental language. It is "died by suicide," "substance use disorder," and "person in recovery," not "committed suicide," "substance abuse," or "addict/drunk/alcoholic." Baby steps.

To those of you struggling:
Courage is facing fear in the midst of vulnerability.
You can do hard things, but you cannot do them alone.
We will show up for you. You can get better. You *will* get better. We want you here.

To all of you:
Put health first. Health is more important than your/their professional success and even their ability to practice medicine.

Don't assume anything. Sometimes the "distance traveled" is clear, most times it is not. Many physicians have had serious traumatic event *prior* to medical training. Be kind to one another.

Mastery is the result of mistakes not perfection. Mastery requires discipline, dedication, and focus. It also requires failure.

Your profession is not your identity. Yes, our work is incredibly meaningful. It is an honor and a privilege to be a surgeon. Define your values and align your goals accordingly. It will make you happier and also a better doctor.

Isolation is the harbinger of grief. Authentic connection is everything. Feel the pain.

Get in the game. Get uncomfortable. Take care of one another.

Cry.

Dr. Cunningham is a fierce advocate for mental health.

I'll Never Float Again

Emily M. Herzberg

There was a singular moment when I became a patient. Lying on a stretcher outside the operating room I waited. The circulator nurse had already taken my glasses relegating me to focus on my own thoughts. I reviewed the events of the prior week. As a first-year neonatology fellow, my weeks were busy, filled with 24-hour calls caring for critically ill newborns, but nothing about my job could have prepared me for that week. The hallway was cold. I looked down at the goose bumps quickly developing on my arms, encircling the 24-gauge IV my team had struggled to place. I closed my eyes and thought back to my recent night shift, the exact moment standing in the clean utility room in the neonatal ICU, when I noticed the blood on my scrubs. It was easy to shrug off. Blood was a routine part of my job. It could have been a remnant from one of the procedures I had completed that shift. But then I noticed it—a mole on my side, a mole that had been there for as long as I could remember, was bleeding. Next thing I knew I was lying on an exam table, still wearing my scrub bottoms, my dermatologist performing a biopsy of the bleeding mole. My rational brain, typically calm under pressure, the same brain that could counsel parents trying to make decisions for their critically ill newborn, was panicking. My thoughts and emotions were racing. Being in medicine I knew instantly that a bleeding mole was a bad sign. I looked up at my dermatologist who was smiling one of those fear-hiding smiles. I felt tears start to well up and despite my best efforts to curtail my emotions, to engage my rational brain, I started to cry. It was at that moment that I became a patient.

Four days later, on a frigid afternoon in February, my dermatologist called to tell me the news: I had stage 3 melanoma. I was walking outside in downtown Boston when I received the call. I held it together just long enough to hang up, and then I crouched in a corner of Newbury Street. Despite the cold, I was surrounded by seemingly happy city-goers sipping their coffee and window-shopping, and yet, I had never been more alone. All the feelings I had felt days earlier came flooding back—the smell of the exam room, the fear-hiding smile, and the taste of my tears. I started crying again, but this time it was a wail, a feeling of control loss like I had never felt before. I didn't know it at that moment, but before that diagnosis, I had been floating. I had been making 10-year plans, thinking about my next big trip, who I would fall in love with. Cancer was something that felt like it happened to others, not to me. That phone call clipped my wings and knocked me out of the sky, straight onto my face. Now, here I was, waiting outside the operating room for my surgeon to remove the mole along with several lymph nodes to prepare me to start a year of adjuvant treatment to prevent recurrence. I would never float again.

My journey and identity living with melanoma over the past 5 years have taught me more than any of my medical training ever could. Being grounded by a cancer diagnosis and recurrence has given me a deep understanding of the importance of hope and how easy it is for that to be taken away. Even as a trainee, prior to my diagnosis, I would often find myself part of a medical team's perseveration in making sure the parents of a critically ill neonate understood the gravity of their child's condition. Looking back on these encounters since my diagnosis, these meetings with families can't help but feel driven by an internal agenda, as if we, the medical team, cannot believe a family understands a likely poor outcome unless they are in tears asking when their baby will die. Most times, it feels like there is no space for hope or seeing the best in a situation. If families are hopeful or smiling or asking for prayers, it just means they don't get it.

However, my own journey has taught me this simply isn't true. Understanding serious illness is nuanced. When I learned that my cancer had progressed to stage 4 with new metastases in my lungs, just 3 years after my initial diagnosis, I remember my immediate, intense feeling of fear. I was scared to die, scared that I wouldn't have the time to make my life mean something. Alongside it, however, I was hopeful. There I was, holding both fear and hope, seemingly contradictory emotions, at the same time. I learned this is both possible and necessary, and it didn't mean that I was in denial regarding my diagnosis. Rather, it was hope, peeking through the cloud of fear that enabled me to wake up the next morning and put my two feet on the floor, walk to the bathroom to brush my teeth, and somehow find the energy to go to work to care for others. Hope gave back to me some sense of control. It's what keeps me from feeling like I did that day in the dermatologist's office or cowering alone in a corner of bustling Newbury Street. This feeling is something that never would have made sense to me before my own diagnosis, but it has made me a better doctor.

Five years later I'm sitting in a stark white office room in the neonatal ICU. A couple is sitting in front of me. They have recently learned their baby has a serious congenital anomaly. As I begin our consultation, I wonder what these parents will remember about this moment. Will it be the paint-stripped walls, evidence of ongoing construction, the faint smell of burnt popcorn wafting from the nurses' break room, or something I haven't yet noticed. Each parent has an uneasy smile—I recognize it instantly, that fear-hiding smile. It's almost as if I can see them falling from the sky as they sit in front of me, their wings being clipped. They might not know it yet, but they will never float again. "Tell me how you feel and how I'm finding you," I say. It's a simple, but powerful question. It's an invitation for families to be their authentic selves. It's a question I wish more people had asked me at the beginning of my journey. The answer could be anything—hopeful, fearful, anxious, content, at peace, or most likely somewhere in between. And then I sit and I listen. I never pretend to have all the answers, but I always make sure families know that I am comfortable with the swirling feeling of contradictory emotions. My own winding journey with cancer has taught me to hold space with my patients and their parents, to help them process the complicated feelings surrounding serious illness, and most importantly, to sit with them while they do so. If I can give anything to the families

I care for, it is the ability to carry this load at their most vulnerable times and to help them find a world where both fear and hope make sense.

> Dr. Herzberg has a particular love for animals, especially her two goldendoodles, Jackson and McKinley. They have been an integral part of her cancer journey, providing lots of snuggles during her most challenging days. She loves traveling with her husband and has recently become a major aficionado of Disney World. In her free time, she enjoys gardening, cooking, and Pure Barre workouts. She has recently taken up writing and is hoping to contribute to more books like this one in the future.

The 7-Year Consult

Rana L. A. Awdish

It's dusk and I'm sitting in the hospital parking structure unable to turn the wheel of my car. Every joint is a detonating bomb, as if an invisible fuse has been ignited and they are imploding in series. Eyes closed, my joints feel outsized and cartoonish, as if they've been hit by a mallet and have ballooned completely out of proportion. Eyes open, I can see that my hands aren't swollen or red. I am annoyed by their uselessness and also because they fail to make the pain visible. To make it real to others.

The severity of this pain is new, though the material fact of the pain is not. I had first sought out a diagnosis when I was still a medical resident in New York. I had fainted in the shower, and that episode, in addition to ongoing fatigue, joint pain, and vague lab abnormalities had led me to the rheumatology clinic at the Hospital for Special Surgery. Despite a comprehensive evaluation and multiple vials of blood analyzed, they could not determine the cause.

"The American College of Rheumatology has criteria for the diagnosis of lupus, which is very specific," the doctor said. He began listing what the criteria were, as if I had asked him a question in an oral exam: "Discoid lesions, malar rash, non-erosive arthritis, pericarditis…."

I nodded, which was intended to indicate that I understood the constraints of his very finite lens. I understood that it wasn't going to be possible to think creatively about my symptoms. There was an agreed-upon set of symptoms in a chart. The chart was the decider, not him. My nod also had the unintentional effect of validating him.

"See, you understand. You don't meet diagnostic criteria, simple as that," he said. I read relief in his demeanor and smiled despite myself.

"This IS good news," the physician said, patting my knee, "you don't want to be sick."

Embarrassment bloomed in my cheeks: *He thought I wanted to be sick.*

I nodded passively and left the exam room with his words rippling through me.

There was something in that casual dismissal that took root. These were the experts, the best in the city, in a city that was the best in the world. The ostensibly good news felt more like being handed a prescription that said, *I, the authority, doubt you and so you should probably start doubting what you know internally because it doesn't match objective, agreed-upon reality.* The roots of that rejection spread deep and wide, tethering me to a skepticism of my own body. If the messages my body sent me were so patently useless, then I would ignore them.

I try moving the gearshift to put the car into reverse, which incites my right shoulder joint. I press the brake, and my knee and ankle shriek. My elbows throb rhythmically, a misplaced heartbeat. The pain stops my breath short. I fear breathing deeply, worried what pain it will trigger, and my mind reads the short breaths as danger, which makes me anxious, quickens my breath and pulse, and begins a restless spiral that's difficult to stop.

I had sought out other opinions. Each time feeling the acute vulnerability of elaborating a list of "complaints" that were not perfectly coherent, not easily categorized. Fatigue, joint pain, hair loss. Easy enough for them to overlay all of it with a psychosomatic fabric, and hand the bundle back to me. Each time accepting someone's professional opinion that there was nothing to label, nothing to treat.

What do you think is going on?
Do you feel depressed?
Are you hoping for a diagnosis?
Fellowship training is hard—of course you are tired.

I was being conditioned to think that communicating about the pain was not useful. That it made people around me uncomfortable, when I placed them in a position of having to refute the experience of my body from a position of authority. I barely even notice when I start to prioritize their comfort over my own and disregard my own lived experience.

I briefly consider leaving the car, before remembering the mechanics of walking. I decided going back inside is impossible. I find a bottle of ibuprofen in my purse and take four with the cold morning coffee in my travel mug. I recline the seat, watch the parking lot empty, and wait for the medicine to work. And it does work. After 2 hours I can reasonably safely drive home. I can collapse in bed. I can claim to have *just had a long day.* I can join everyone in minimizing the symptoms.

I will eventually start taking ibuprofen or other anti-inflammatory medications around the clock. I will take enough to erode my stomach's protective lining. I will discover this when I vomit blood in an airplane bathroom, on a flight back from a medical conference in Wisconsin. I will go straight from the airport to having an endoscopy. I will be told to stop taking ibuprofen. This will force me back into the exam room of yet another rheumatologist.

This time it's different. I cannot present my symptoms impassively and pretend to be ok for the sake of anyone's comfort. The one thing that had helped me to get through my days has been taken away and has been blamed for causing even bigger problems. She enters the exam room and I start to cry almost immediately.

She dips her head down, to catch my downward gaze and nods. Her whole presence is warm, with chestnut hair and soft features. Her eyes track my distress, and her face mirrors mine at times. I explain the pain, apologizing and offering her exit ramps, not wanting to coerce a diagnosis out of pity or ambivalence, or a need to escape the mess of me. I wait for the slightest suggestion of frustration or apathy. I find neither. She is affirming and unshakable in her presence. She leans in, she does not interrupt. Eventually I stop.

"It sounds like you've been suffering for a long time," she says and stands.

I nod, grateful for the acknowledgment.

"Some of my colleagues have dismissed you," she offers, examining my joints one by one.

I nod again, and shrug apologetically. I worry that I'm now putting her not only in a position of refuting my lived experience and concerns but also of possibly contradicting her colleagues.

She shakes her head, sits back down and sighs. She spreads the round hem of her skirt so that it's evenly distributed around her. She smooths the pleats gently, as she chooses her words.

"These diagnoses are not set in stone, and there is a lot that we don't know. You've told me enough to think that we should try treating you as though this is an autoimmune connective tissue disease, which it probably is, even if we can't give it a neatly perfect label and tie it with a bow. You don't need me to tell you that these diseases disproportionately affect women, and Medicine's not great at listening to us, really."

We could try to treat it.

"And, if you feel better on treatment, well that's its own kind of confirmation, isn't it?" she says. She shrugs, as if to say, *I may not know everything exactly right now, but we'll figure it out.*

I nod and feel lightened by a kind of tenuous optimism.

She suggests a medication and elaborates on possible side effects, not realizing, in my desperation, I could have been convinced to try a solution of turpentine mixed with lead. I find the simple act of being listened to and having my suffering validated to be healing, independent even of any treatment.

From the onset of the symptoms to initiation of therapy took roughly 7 years. A time lapse that existed despite all of my very real privilege and access, and all of the self-advocacy and awareness I could bring to each encounter.

Seven years door to door.

Dr. Awdish is the author of *In Shock*, a critically acclaimed, bestselling memoir based on her own critical illness. She has sought to integrate communication skills training, visual thinking strategies, and narrative medicine into the curriculum for faculty and trainees. She believes in the power of art to heal and creates both visual art and narrative nonfiction essays.

Joy Machine

Emily Silverman

I was tired of bringing my heating pad to work—people asked questions—so I bought a pack of hand warmers on Amazon, the kind you keep in your ski jacket pockets, only I kept them in my white coat pockets, occasionally stuffing one down my pants while nobody was looking in an attempt to soothe the pain.

Imagine the nerves in your bladder firing, sending an urgent message to your brain—*you have to pee, now*—and then you sit down in the bathroom but nothing comes out. I felt that almost every day for over a year, and it nearly drove me mad.

I was also waking up in the middle of the night, feeling as though someone were wringing the blood out of my pelvis—a pain so intense I couldn't hold a conversation. Boaz told me to count to 50, and we did, together, until the ibuprofen kicked in.

I asked two different gynecologists if I might have endometriosis, but both said it was unlikely, since my bladder symptoms were so prominent, and since my cramps were worse when I was on the pill than when I was off. "Then what is causing my pain?" I asked. "Maybe it's some kind of nerve pain?" one doctor said. "Residency is stressful," another doctor said. "Plus, you're planning a wedding."

I knew the pain wasn't from stress or planning a wedding, but I wanted to be a good patient, so I agreed to try meditation and physical therapy, even though I was about to start a month-long cardiology rotation, during which I would have only 4 days off, and work a 28-hour shift every fourth night.

During one shift, there was a lull in the work, so I found the call room—a closet-sized chamber with a cot and computer—and lay down, desperate for sleep. My bladder was alive with discomfort. I tossed and turned in the cot, its metal haunches whining and crackling under my weight. I put a hand warmer down my pants, but it quickly slid through a leg-hole. I went to the bathroom. Peed a little. Got back in the cot, my bladder still tight like a fist.

Gradually, my thoughts slowed down, coalescing and separating like blobs of oil. I tasted the sweet nectar of REM—for 18 minutes, and then my pager erupted in beeps. I jerked awake, adrenaline squirting into my blood. I checked the pager. A new patient. I slid on my clogs and went back to work.

At home, the following morning, the muscles of my pelvis were contracted as if around a wound. I swayed, fighting off the vertigo of sleep deprivation, and then started to cry, sitting on the toilet with my scrubs down around my ankles. There was no way out of this. No YES or NO button that appeared, with a message asking, "Do you want to continue?" My heart kept beating; my nerves kept firing; my kidneys filtered blood; my liver dribbled bile; my head hurt; my feet stank.

"Come to bed," Boaz said, standing in the doorway. He helped me over. Held me against his chest. His body felt dense and warm. I loved his smell.

Boaz worked at an education technology startup and part of his job was creating spreadsheets. He was good at it, and actually kind of liked it. He'd even created a spreadsheet to track our monthly spending, whose cells changed values based on other cells' values, according to algorithms he had written.

He opened a fresh spreadsheet. He called it "Joy Machine."

He typed:

Hi, sweety. You're in a funk. First:
AVOID sitting in the bathroom.
AVOID internet wormholes.

Then:

Reload page (Cmd + R) to find out what activity you'll be doing.

It was like a digital Magic 8-ball, with dozens of suggestions. Here are some examples:

Play guitar.
Draw something.
Shop online.
Call a friend.
Learn about something new.

I hit Cmd + R. A message popped up. It said: *"Read part of a book."*
I did.
Ten minutes later, I was asleep.

Months later, the pain came again in the middle of the night. I shook Boaz awake and moved to the bathroom—but this time, it wasn't our dinky bathroom, whose showerhead squirted water over the middle, not the side, of the tub. It was a huge, marble bathroom with a Jacuzzi. We were in Miami, Florida, and it was the night before our wedding.

"Sorry I woke you," I said.

"Always wake me," he said. I thought I might vomit from the pain. We counted.

The next day, he married me. I was worried he wouldn't. This problem was new, and neither of us knew what the future held.

Months later, a new pain appeared in the left side of my pelvis. What was it? A hernia? I went for an ultrasound.

"I don't see anything," the ultrasound tech said.

"It must be there," I told her. She scanned again.

"I think I found it," she said. I was thrilled. An answer!

But then I saw a respected surgeon who examined me and the ultrasound images, and told me that there was no hernia there.

The sticking feeling on my left side continued to worsen. I kept peeing, not peeing, waking up with cramps. I cried often, feeling depleted and alien to myself. I felt as if my situation would never change. That it meant the end of my medical career, my relationships, and my life.

"Use the Joy Machine," Boaz said.

Take a bath.
Order and eat some comfort food, unless not hungry.
Write something.

I was on the floor of my apartment rolling around on an orange—the physical therapist's prescription—when I decided it was time for someone to cut me open. I found a surgeon who would do it, but she was about to leave the country for 3 weeks on a medical mission trip. We scheduled the operation for the week she got back. I kept working; I kept getting worse.

Do deep breathing exercises.
Count objects, like body parts, or things in the room.
Put things in perspective: watch or read something about the universe.

Finally, the day of the surgery came. Boaz and my friend Elizabeth brought me to the same hospital at which I worked. I shielded my face in the pre-op waiting room, hoping nobody would recognize me. Behind a curtain, I changed into an inflatable purple hospital gown and a bouffant cap.

"You look cute," Boaz said.

Afterward, I woke up to find Boaz and Elizabeth at my bedside. They told me I'd had endometriosis all over my bladder and left ovary, and that the surgeon had removed it. I kept forgetting, because of the anesthesia. They kept telling me.

Meanwhile, they wheeled an old man into the empty space next door. His big toe was wrapped up, like a gauzy ice cream cone. I recognized him; I had been his doctor 2 days ago on the inpatient medicine consult service. "What floor is his room on?" one nurse asked another. "Thirteen," I said, groggy.

When we got home, the fridge was full of ginger ale. Boaz set up a plate with saltine crackers, and made sure I took my pain medicine on time. A few days later, I was ready to see the pictures from the surgery. My pink glistening insides and a silver probe, pushing things this way and that.

Dr. Silverman is the creator and host of the award-winning medical storytelling program, *The Nocturnists*. Her writing has been supported by MacDowell and The Pulitzer Center and published in *The New York Times*, *Boston Globe*, *Virginia Quarterly Review*, and more.

Free Refills

Peter Grinspoon

One wintery afternoon, in February 2005, I waddled back to my office from a lunchtime lecture, sponsored by Big Pharm, which left me in equal parts sleepy and full. I was intending to continue working my way through the endless problems of my waiting patients in our hectic primary care clinic. It is difficult to find the words to describe how flabbergasted I was to find the Drug Enforcement Agency and the state police waiting for me in my office, like a hostile trap that had been set. I tried to engage them in polite conversation, trying to buy time to make sense out of their incongruous presence. They cut me short, "doc, cut the crap, we know you've been writing bad scripts." It went sharply downhill from there.

The officers instructed me that three felony prescription violations were outstanding, having to do with some highly dubious prescriptions I had written. They instructed me to show up at the courthouse the next morning for fingerprinting. They were quite unfriendly, even bullying, but at least they were courteous enough not to arrest me in front of my patients and my staff.

What tripped me up was a prescription I had written for the powerful opioid painkiller named Vicodin. I had written this in the name of our former nanny, who had long since left the country. In my addicted brain, which was desperate to maintain its access to prescription opioids, it had occurred to me to continue writing prescriptions for her and picking them up for my own use for months after she had departed the country. The pharmacist eventually became suspicious and phoned me to confirm her doubts. When I couldn't verify my own birthdate, it became quite obvious to her that I wasn't who I was pretending to be. She would have been justified in calling the show "America's Dumbest Criminals" where I surely would have been awarded a leading role. Instead, she called the police.

Truth be told, I had become profoundly addicted to prescription painkillers over the previous 10 years. I had been using opioids to medicate away the emotional distress that I felt, first as an overworked medical student, then as a medical resident, and finally as a physician newly minted into practice. The additional stresses of new fatherhood and a surreally hostile marital situation were only compounded by long work hours and sleep deprivation. I had discovered that a small handful of Vicodin made all of this misery disappear, if only for a few hours. It was ecstatic, at least at first. As my addiction progressed, I needed daily pills to forestall the soul-crushing opioid withdrawal symptoms.

I never got high on the job, though I suspect this was a line I would have eventually crossed if my descent into addiction weren't so rudely—though fortuitously—interrupted. As it were, it is fair to say that I was rarely close to my personal best while caring for patients. There's something about staying up all night snorting Oxycontin or spending your entire workday in shaking agonies of withdrawal, that inhibits you from putting in your most compassionate and conscientious effort.

The felony charges that were filed by the police unleashed a firestorm of excruciating consequences in my life. The medical board effectively suspended my medical license—it took me more than 3 years to get it back. I was sentenced to 2 years of supervised probation with a garrulous but paranoid probation officer, whom I had to visit in the basement of our dingy local courthouse every week, along with the other criminals. I wasn't allowed to leave the state without permission. I ended up living back with my elderly parents, unable to consistently visit with my two small children.

Out of options, out of a job, stripped of many of my credentials, and out of any say in my immediate future plans, I was railroaded into attending 90 days of rehab. I went to a facility that purportedly specializes in treating addicted healthcare professionals, though this, like so many other aspects of rehab, turned out to be utter nonsense. I was so opposed to the idea of rehab that they practically had to drag me, with my fingernails clawing the floor. Sartre said hell is other people, but for me, it was being remanded to what I, at the time, perceived to be a 12-step religious cult. I left my stay in rehab with the feeling, which persists to this date, that rehab simply isn't an effective way to treat addiction. Not enough science and too much voodoo and superstition, and too many platitudes, such as "let go and let God." (I still don't know what that means, even though we repeated it daily.)

Medical professionals are at exceedingly high risk for addiction to drugs and alcohol, as well as for other mental health problems, including suicide. The high addiction risk is due to a toxic combination of the stress we are under, toiling away in a broken and exploitative system, and the ready access we have to prescription medications—"free refills." For doctors, it is a perfect storm of stress and access.

The one good thing I can say about rehab is that, while there, I was treated as if I had a disease that needed to be addressed with compassion and empathy (even if the treatment was exceedingly flaky). This was new to me and filled me with hope for the future—perhaps others would understand what I was going through as an unintentional process, beyond my control. It helped prevent me from being overcome by my guilt, by my shame, and by the remorse I had for destroying my life, and for letting down my family, my friends, my colleagues and my patients.

After rehab, when I re-entered the "real" world, I had the profound shock of dealing with both the criminal justice system and the medical board. Both of these institutions treated me not with an iota of compassion, but as if I were a willful malfeasant who had deliberately broken laws for the sake of hedonistic pursuits. This does not represent a modern understanding of addiction. The punishments they meted out were not supportive of my recovery.

One would think that the medical board, an entity composed of doctors, which frequently deals with this common and deadly issue, would understand addiction as a medical disease, and not as a moral failing. In some ways, the medical board was less understanding about addiction than my probation officer, or even my attorney, who, after learning of a flunked drug test, soon after my bust, screamed at me, "you are a major-league screw-up." This hurt my feelings at a cost of $400 dollars an hour. In reality, most people do not go magically from "addicted" to "recovered" without some slips—this is the natural history of addiction.

What ultimately helped me the most in terms of entering and staying in recovery were two things: the ongoing support of the Massachusetts Physician Health Service (PHS), which is part of the Massachusetts Medical Society, and the fact that no one gave up on me. My family, friends, colleagues—they all continued to believe in me.

The PHS is a nonprofit group that supports physicians in recovery, as well as physicians with other problems such as depression and bipolar disorder. PHS counseled, monitored, and drug tested me for years, until I could reasonably demonstrate a solid record of recovery to the medical board regarding, and could thus petition them for a return to medical practice. Importantly, they provided vital peer support which sustained my spirits. Over a 7-year period, I provided 400 drug tests, which comes out to about 20 gallons of urine. I believe that the long-term follow-up was essential to my ability to enter into sustained recovery because addiction is a chronic disease that requires long-term care just as do any other chronic conditions, such as diabetes or hypertension.

They treated me with a harsh version of "contingency management," which is a modality of treatment where they offer rewards or punishments for staying free of drugs. Typically, one offers a reward to patients who are addicted to not consume drugs. If they provide a urine sample that is free of any drugs of misuse, they might receive cash. Contingency management has been shown to be effective.

I was given a more brutal type of contingency management which involved punishments not rewards: flunk any more drug tests and you'll never get your medical license back. This is not a "warm and fuzzy" way to treat anyone, it doesn't really comport with the natural history of addiction, and the stress involved probably gave me PTSD. But, it worked. I have been in recovery now for 15 years and counting. I have been back practicing medicine successfully—or at least creditably given how utterly broken and dysfunctional our system is, for 14 years.

In truth, the one thing that PHS, and the medical board, did very wrong is they never offered me Suboxone (buprenorphine), the medication which, along with methadone, results in at least a 50% decrease in deaths from overdose. Through this neglect, they put my life in danger and, essentially, committed—or, forced my doctors to commit—malpractice. They historically have shunned these medications because they think it "impairs" doctors, even though there is absolutely no evidence for this. Recently, they have been beaten senseless on this particular issue, by articles in the *New England Journal of Medicine* and editorials on *NPR*'s "All Things Considered," and now they say they provide Suboxone on a case-by-case basis, rather than blanketly prohibiting it.

Having returned to the clinical practice of primary care, now that I was in recovery from addiction, I no longer take being a doctor for granted. I view it more as a privilege than an entitlement.

Many of the qualities that one needs to get into recovery in the first place are the same qualities that are sought out in our most popular and effective doctors: empathy, mindfulness, gratitude, and humility. For having suffered through all of my struggles, I am a better listener, more patient, and less likely to be judgmental or oblivious than I was 15 years ago. I spend less time worrying about all of the things that can go wrong, and which are out of my control, and I am much more focused on the present moment. This is a gift to doctor and patient alike.

In 2013, I was hired as an associate director by the same PHS, in order to leverage my experience, strength, and hope to help physicians overcome their addictions and to address the chaos that their addictions were causing in their own lives. I sat at the same long brown wooden table, only this time on the other side. It was a much more comfortable vantage point than it had been 8 years earlier. I feel uniquely equipped to help these struggling physicians because of the painful lessons that I had learned.

With appropriate help, physicians have a relatively high recovery rate from addiction, though given how taboo this subject is, and how confidential treatment is, we don't have accurate data. Recovery is by no means guaranteed, and I know several physicians that have died by overdose, several that are homeless, and many that never managed to return to medicine. Generally, physicians encounter a relatively high degree of success in part because we have so much to lose, such as our hard-earned livelihoods and identities, and in part because we have financial resources to throw at medical care, therapy, drug tests, aftercare, peer support, and the other necessary components of a strong recovery program. In my case, it definitely helped that I was white and middle class—an ugly truth about our criminal justice system, which affords some categories of people more of a second chance than others.

It is imperative that we find ways to export or emulate this model for success for people suffering from substance misuse in other walks of life, so that we can maximize the number of people that can return to productive, meaningful lives. This could prevent thousands of needless deaths as well. Policymakers need to understand that there is no quick fix for addiction, and that people need long-term support. We need to fund the infrastructure to follow people from their acute detoxification all the way, for several years, until they are in stable recovery. We need to provide the medications for addiction that are proving to be so profoundly effective, such as Suboxone. People need to be provided a credible pathway out of addiction, which includes safe housing, jobs training, and affordable healthcare.

As it stands, a minority of patients suffering from addiction gets adequate treatment. Providing the necessary resources to support, to uplift, and to follow those who are struggling from substance misuse is the ethical thing to do. It would also would save billions of dollars in the long run. It would make us a healthier and more cohesive society as a whole.

Dr. Grinspoon is the author of Seeing Through the Smoke: A Cannabis Specialist Untangles the Truth About Marijuana *and* Free Refills: A Doctor Confronts His Addiction.

Doctors Are Humans: Breaking Painful Stereotypes

Giuseppina Romano-Clarke

The day before I was scheduled to take my MCAT exam, I was diagnosed with multiple sclerosis. The specialist I was seeing did not have time to wait for my husband to join me at the appointment. After a review of my tests and a physical examination he simply said, "You have a demyelinating disease, you know, MS." While I was relieved to find the reason for the fatigue and strange feelings in my hands and legs that I had experienced for a few months, I sat stunned and alone trying to reconcile multiple sclerosis with my pursuit of a career in medicine. I had an uncle with the disease who was confined to a wheelchair in his 40s. This was a terrifying future to contemplate. I was 27 years old, had been in the United States for 3 years, was married, and had an active toddler son. Getting into medical school and completing the training was going to be hard even before having to deal with this new challenge. Should I reconsider my career plans?

Becoming a doctor had been my purpose since I was 5 years old, when I had a tonsillectomy because of frequent episodes of streptococcal pharyngitis. On the day of the surgery, screaming in fear they took me away from my parents. The operating room was dark except for the blinding lights of the surgical field. While a nurse held me tightly in his lap, the surgeon used a metal instrument to keep my mouth open, sprayed a numbing medicine in my throat, and snipped out my tonsils. I could feel the blood dripping down my throat and the urine running down my pants. The postoperative popsicles they gave me and the coloring books that people brought me when they visited were little consolation. The pain, the fear, and the embarrassment I had experienced was intense and unforgettable. I did not want any other child to go through what had happened to me. I was on a mission. I was going to become a pediatrician!

My commitment to becoming a doctor matured in my adolescent years during volunteer work with the Red Cross. The images of an elderly woman infested with lice lying alone in a hospital bed, the financial strain on a family of a girl with cerebral palsy whose mother had to quit her job to become her main caregiver, and the agony of a mother who lost her baby during the devastating 1980 earthquake in Naples when the roof of her decrepit house fell on his crib were hard to forget.

I realized that health and disease need should be placed into the context of real people who have a broad range of needs and life circumstances. I understood that my traumatic tonsillectomy was a result of the narrow-minded focus on performing the procedure efficiently without considering the impact it may have had on my psychological well-being. It was clear to me that to be a good doctor one had to have a deep understanding of the human being behind a patient. I was ready to embrace this challenge.

My path to becoming a doctor did not follow a straight line. I started medical school in Italy but moved to Boston in my early 20s after meeting my husband, Jack. I found a job in a lab to keep my connection with medicine and to help make ends meet, and I signed up for college classes to complete the requirements to apply to an American medical school. Jack and I did not come from well-off families, so the early years of my life in this country were not easy. We had many breakfasts of homemade popcorn and dinners of tortilla chips and salsa from the pub where Jack was working as a bartender. I worked full time doing medical research during the day, went to Harvard extension at night, and became a mother.

Then, there was my diagnosis of multiple sclerosis. It was a terrible shock, but I was not going to let it stop me from doing what I wanted in my personal and professional lives. I believed that my experiences as a patient and a volunteer in Italy and my recent diagnosis of a chronic disease gave me a clearer sense of what it was like to be at the other end of the stethoscope. This was going to be as important to my education as a doctor as the technical training that I would receive in medical school. On the outside, I seemed strong and determined. However, behind the strong façade, as I was pushing myself to give the best in everything I was doing, I was battling with insecurity and gnawing self-denigration. In the competitive world of American medicine, training and practice required mental and physical prowess and a single-minded dedication to the profession. I was afraid that I was not going to make the cut.

When I applied to medical school in 1993, I did not disclose my multiple sclerosis diagnosis since my disease was invisible at that point. Here I was, already an older student, with a family, and born in a foreign country. I did not fit the stereotype engrained in the medical culture. Having multiple sclerosis was going to be viewed for sure as an additional liability. What I experienced confirmed my reservations. In fact, a medical student with whom I spoke during one of my selection interviews asked me how I was planning to juggle family and medical school. After my acceptance to medical school, I was invited to participate in an orientation before classes that was offered to a group of "untraditional" students based on their racial-ethnic backgrounds and place of birth. Although well-intended, we had been labeled as vulnerable even before having a chance to prove ourselves.

I struggled to fit in during my residency as well. When my father had a serious post-operative complication, I absolutely needed to go back to Italy. I had been afraid to ask for the time off to go for the surgery because no one in my prestigious Boston pediatric residency program had taken a personal leave. My resident colleagues seemed consumed by work and career. Or, more likely, there were others who like me were struggling with keeping a healthy work-life balance. There was just no space to talk about it. We were all expected to be superhumans that could cruise through sleep deprivation with grace and still deliver at peak performance. I was able to take a leave for my father's medical emergency, but once his illness extended longer than expected, I was pressured to come back to meet my responsibility as a resident. I did not dare to say that my family was as important to me as my career. I also kept to myself the fact that, on the breaks from spending time in the ICU with my dad, I was receiving infusions of high-dose steroids for the optic neuritis I developed because of the extreme stress I was encountering. Ironically, once I was back in Boston, I was assigned to the pediatric ICU, a chilling reminder of what I had just left behind. Because of my medical background, I had been the only family member the hospital had allowed access into my dad's ICU room. He died alone a week after I came back to Boston, something that brings tears to my eyes to this day as I think about the isolation he may have felt during the last moments of his life.

I have been a pediatrician for 25 years and I love my job as much as I expected, maybe even more! I spent the first 15 years of my career working in Dorchester and Chelsea, Massachusetts, two communities known for their racial and ethnic diversity and health and socioeconomic disparities. While I deeply enjoyed caring for individual patients, I had my eyes set on changing systems to improve their care. For example, when my young patients had devastating oral disease due to prolonged bottle feeding and there were no dentists accepting to see them, I worked at the local, state, and national levels to promote the inclusion of preventive oral health services in routine pediatric visits. I kept true to my holistic view of medical practice by doing home visits to see children whose families had transportation issues, attending school meetings to advocate for services for my patients with learning disabilities when their parents did not speak English, and delivering food, clothes, and furniture when they were needed.

I left primary care for personal reasons, and I have worked in the Newborn Unit at Massachusetts General Hospital for the past 10 years. Despite receiving several awards for my medical and teaching efforts, the undercurrent of self-questioning remained alive and well, fueled by the worsening of my ability to walk. After a few embarrassing falls, I had to resign myself to using a walker for long distances. As a result, I was stopped on my way to the hospital lobby when using the employees' entrance. Once more I was coming up short in terms of expectations and I was not fitting in with the stereotypical image of a doctor.

In an essay about art and medicine published in the *Lancet* in 2009, the authors suggested, "The most dramatic learning for medical trainees and physicians can come when it is a peer who has a disability, rather than a patient." In fact, two female medical students I worked with a few years ago provided me with the greatest lesson in self-acceptance. One of the students was in a wheelchair due to a car accident when she was 9 years old. The other shared with me that she had multiple sclerosis. Both students were smart, strong, and courageous young women who were pursuing a combined M.D.–Ph.D. from Harvard Medical School. They were not just my trainees. They were my peers. It was easy for me to talk to them about my experience as a doctor with a disability without being afraid of judgment. I felt a profound admiration for them, and I had an epiphany! I realized that I had many of their positive attributes. I could finally look at myself with compassion and appreciate my accomplishments rather than wasting energy on what external pressures had made me feel were my shortcomings. Doctors are humans. They have strengths and weaknesses and *that is ok*. Their value should be measured by their passion for lifelong learning and the heart and soul that they put into caring for their patients rather than in fitting into a specific mold. I share this pearl with the trainees with whom I work when I am on service at the hospital. It helps me as a reminder that I am not an impostor, it helps my students and residents to focus on growing as humans and physicians rather than worrying about performance, and I hope it may help you as well in times of self-questioning.

> Dr. Romano-Clarke's career focuses on healthcare quality improvement and addressing health disparities. She spent 15 years as a pediatrician in Dorchester and Chelsea, Massachusetts, then 13 years as a hospitalist in the Massachusetts General Hospital Newborn Nursery, where she was the Director of Medical Education and Director of Breastfeeding Quality Improvement. When she is not busy with work, Dr. Romano-Clarke loves spending time at the beach and cooking Italian meals for her family and friends.

A Journey's Journal: Finding Strength in Words and Gratitude in Experience

David V. Diamond

Just after sundown, as the red bag of stem cells were dripping into my body, my wife, two of my children, my brother and his wife, the Rabbi and two nurses from the BMT team gathered around my bed, all with purple gloves and surgical masks on. The Rabbi guided us individually to reflect on how we felt about the healing taking place. Then he asked my daughter if she would like to sing a song. I could see she was barely holding back tears above her mask. She was surprised and probably did not feel she could perform on cue, and yet I sensed she knew I would love it. After a pause of several moments, she said, "I have a song," and began... "The sun will come out tomorrow...." Her notes were on-key, airy soft, but heavy with emotion. When she finished, we joined hands, and the Rabbi said a prayer in English and Hebrew offering healing and well-being. It was a moment, and the spirit was with us.

When the infusion finished, one by one all left the room. It was the evening shift, and I was alone now. New life was flowing through my heart, a memory of what had just happened was etched on my soul, and there was the illumination of love glowing in the quiet of my room.

For the last 6 months, we had been preparing for that day, ever since that first abnormal blood count report popped so unexpectedly onto my clinical computer screen at MIT. Six months of preparation for when my brother's 10.9 million well-matched stem cells were infused, hopefully to find their new home engrafted in my bones. It would be a few weeks before we would know that the procedure worked, but as of then we were on a successful course. My brother had managed to pump out twice the required cells needed, a good prognostic indicator!

People ask, as a doctor who experienced a life-threatening illness and its dangerous treatment, do you have a new perspective on life or medicine? I consider this question anew each time it is asked, and I come to the same conclusion: no. Not having had a transformative experience from such suffering is, honestly, a bit disappointing. Having gone through a very difficult regimen of chemotherapy, bone marrow transplant, and months of recovery, I might have hoped for a redeeming epiphany or a "silver lining." But no, I repeatedly find on reflection that I am the same person, with the same appreciation of life and its meaning, the same realistic opinion of medical care, as before my surprise diagnosis of advanced myelodysplastic syndrome. What has emerged though is a more explicit written expression of who I am and how I am experiencing this life challenge. The form this has taken is an online journal on the website CaringBridge. Doing this was a suggestion of a Dana Farber Cancer Institute social worker my wife and I met with during the acute phase of my treatment. As an example, the opening paragraphs of this essay were extracted from one entry.

During my journey and journaling, I have found comfort in reflecting with a wider perspective, often inspired by Nature. For example, I made this entry one evening about a year after my transplant, while on the Rhode Island shore viewing a dramatic summer storm for nearly an hour.

Huge, brilliant flashes illuminated the distant sky over Block Island Sound as bursts of lightning flashed from towering cloud to cloud and occasionally pierced down to the horizon in bright orange bolts. Then came the booming cracks of thunder and pounding sheets of wind-driven rain. Despite my wife's fears and admonition to move away from the large sliding glass door, I felt safe from the powerful storm. I did however appreciate how people could imagine that such a heavenly display was evidence of celestial beings with fearful and transcendental powers. As a rational modern man, I do not share such beliefs and yet I did experience this awesome sight as extraordinary and a powerful challenge to our presumptive sense of control in our world. The sun rises, the moon goes through phases, the tides and the seasons change. Nature proceeds predictably and silently and is routinely unnoticed. But a thunderstorm is sudden, unpredictable, loudly threatening and commands our attention. It brings with it uncertainty and fear. It is a reminder of Nature's true mystery.

So it is with one's health. We are born, we grow, we mature, we age, predictably and silently. Our cuts heal, our minor illnesses come and go, a good night's sleep treats most aches and pains. All quietly miraculous, really. Then suddenly something changes, an accident, a serious illness, a genetic weakness breaks through, and we face a fearsome uncertainty. We seek to understand, look for causes and reasons, but find no simple answers. We reach for the way to regain control and return to normalcy. With the best of medical care, and some luck (and a prayer), we hopefully regain the routine of health. Yet once beyond the darkness, do we remember the storm, the brilliant flashes and thunderous claps that threatened us in the night?

I have been very lucky. I have survived for 4 years despite the odds, due to a combination of luck, superb medical care, generous medical insurance coverage, family and community support, financial security, and some personal effort. Who knows what health challenges lie ahead for me? I am still under treatment for moderate graft-versus-host disease and at risk for infections, and other issues.

However, I have found resources that give me confidence I can weather any storm. One of these is my inner voice, which can speak through my writing, giving me comfort and strength. Other sources of strength have been observing Nature and being supported by my community. For in Nature, I saw that though the seasons change and with it life cycles. There is a dependable permanence and wonderful rebirth. In my community of family and friends developed over years, I found a depth of love and support that cannot be appreciated until it rises up and embraces you during a crisis. After every entry in my journal, I received numerous words of support sent to my journal, by email, by phone, and often in person. My main support, my wife of now 32 years, was always at my side, keeping me safe and nurturing me, along with my four adult children. And they, in turn, were supported by their friends both in words and deeds.

The challenge of death has brought forth the vitality of my life and an appreciation of the world that surrounds me. So maybe, I have been in a way transformed by my illness. Maybe I have had an epiphany after all. I have not changed, but I have discovered my true self, within Nature and in community. For this, despite all, I am grateful.

Due to my illness, its treatment, and added particular risk for me of the COVID-19 epidemic, I have retired from active medical practice. I still keep up my continuing medical education learning, occasionally attending virtual grand rounds, and keep an Up-To-Date subscription. I have an expanding practice as what I have come to call my "Friends and Family" medical consultant. I think those folks reaching out to me for guidance not only appreciate the wisdom that I have from 40 years of general medical practice but also perhaps value the fact that I have experienced the personal challenge of a life-threatening illness. Many also have read my journal entries and have found comfort in my personal reflections and underlying optimism despite the initial poor prognosis. They look not only for practical advice on diagnosis and treatment but also for the comfort of reassurance. So although I feel I am the same clinician I have always been, perhaps I have become more of a healer in the deepest sense. Namely, my words now empower my "patients" both with knowledge, and with grace. In this sense, I am a better physician, and, for this, I am also grateful.

> Dr. Diamond has maintained his medical license and has an informal practice where he helps friends and family, including his 97-year-old mother, navigate health concerns and the care system. He also keeps busy organizing educational conferences for his specialty organization, the New England College of Occupational and Environmental Medicine. Personally, he is occupied being the father of four grown children, including mentoring the youngest, a third-year medical student, and as of this summer, being a grandfather.

Lessons Learned

Evonne Kaplan-Liss

One day, in 2012, I woke up in a recovery room at the Mount Sinai Hospital in New York City and instinctively looked down at my stomach. I was woozy, though no more than usual. I'd had 21 abdominal surgeries in the 30 years since I was diagnosed with ulcerative colitis as a teenager. The objective nearly every time had not been to treat my disease or excise something malignant but to avoid the thing I thought I was seeing now through the post-op haze.

"Is that a bag?" I called over to the nursing station, my voice raspy and incredulous.

"Yeah, it's a bag," a nurse replied.

I felt a deep heaviness in my chest. This wasn't supposed to happen, I thought—not now. But it wasn't the ileostomy bag itself that was hard for me to accept. It was that my long fight to avoid it was over—abruptly and seemingly without warning. I had my first surgery when I was 15 and now was 46 when I heard the nurse nonchalantly utter those words. I'd spent most of my adolescence and my entire adult life in this mindset that I should always opt for doing whatever could be done to keep from having a bag. It was the one thing that would make me better but at a cost the adults around me considered too high: the removal of my colon, and in its place a bag.

"Nobody wanted that for a 15-year-old girl," I heard my doctors say. "How's she gonna get married and have kids with a bag?" At my first surgery, my parents felt fortunate that I would have a top surgical team performing what they were told was a "state-of-the-art" procedure—"the Rolls Royce" of gastrointestinal operations. They wondered how many times this procedure had been performed on someone so young and asked to speak to some other parents. But my health declined quickly, and there wasn't time. There were ongoing complications from the start and over 30 years whatever problems came up surgery was always the answer. And I always came out without a bag. Until … "Yeah, it's a bag." So, matter-of-fact.

I remember waking up later in my hospital room in 2012 consumed with my loss but at the same time understanding how my surgeons must be feeling about the results. After all, by this point, I'm not just a chronic patient but also a physician and I've walked in their shoes. I knew how much they cared and how hard it would be for them to face me. I broke the ice in a text to one of my surgeons: "Don't worry. I will be okay." He texted back: "I'm so glad you're taking this in stride. This is one of the worst days of my career."

It felt like days before my surgeons came to see me. My mother was angry. Why, after 21 surgeries, did my surgeon *call her* from the operating room to tell her about the bag rather than breaking the news face to face like he always did? A medical student who held my hand as I went to sleep for what was to be my last surgery appeared in my room later that day. "What happened in there?" I asked her. She replied, "They tried their best to save it. It felt like there was a death in the room. They felt that they failed you." One of the surgeons had cried. And there we have it. My fight against the bag was also my surgeons' fight and we all felt defeated. I knew they did their best, and I felt their love. But I can't help but wonder if I weren't also a physician if I could have understood this dynamic. I may instead have felt angry and neglected, as my mother felt.

A few days after being discharged home, my son Josh saw me crying. He was taken aback, as I never cried after the 20 previous surgeries. "You're just a mother with a bag," he assured me. As it turned out, he was right. Life after the bag was much easier. When I went to my first post-op appointment, I was embarrassed to tell my surgeon how much easier life was abandoning the "Rolls Royce" and going with the "Buick"—as we came to refer to the bag. Like a Buick, without fancy bells and whistles, it was *reliable* and *worked well*. My surgeon responded, "That's what all my patients say that have been through what you have been through."

Another matter-of-fact response, but this time, the shock of it led me to question whether all those surgeries to avoid a bag were the right thing to do. It was the kind of question that can be applied to medical situations of all kinds, for both doctors and their patients: When is enough *enough*?

It was a moment that triggered a search to understand my long and torturous medical life—not only the things that befell me but the choices I'd made and the role my doctors played in those decisions. And now I saw it not just through the lens of a perennial patient but as a journalist and doctor myself.

In high school, I dreamed of becoming a physician. Despite missing the last 2 years, I was discharged from one of my hospital stays just to attend my prom and I even managed to graduate. My health made my future uncertain and prevented me from committing to the rigorous pre-med path. I chose to major in journalism instead, my other passion. I received my degree in journalism from Northwestern University and then landed my first job for Ted Koppel and Nightline. Though I was already making my way in journalism, still burning inside of me was my desire to become a physician. After deep reflection, I left my journalism career behind and applied to medical school. Armed with communication skills honed as a journalist, I was now poised to achieve my "big dream"—to be a physician that trains other doctors to communicate with compassion.

It wasn't until medical school that I realized how sick I had been and appreciated the uncertainty of my future. I gave birth to my oldest son in my third year while living with the complications of yet another "state-of-the-art" procedure we referred to as the "Cadillac"—a step-down from the "Rolls Royce." Surgery to me was like getting an oil change in my car. It was just another thing to do to keep things running smoothly. My first years at the Mount Sinai School of Medicine, at the same hospital where I had been a patient, were a return to familiar surroundings but with a key to the kingdom. I was excited that I could finally communicate with doctors in their mother tongue. But I quickly began to feel I was losing my own life lessons in the process and needed to find a way to stay grounded as a patient and as a doctor. My journalism training came in handy. In the clinic, I instinctively knew the right questions to ask and in a way that showed my empathy and concern for what patients were going through. I didn't have to be taught this. I lived it.

When I began working directly with patients in my third year, I connected many of the routine problems I saw to failures in communication between the healthcare team and patients. I heard doctors throwing medical jargon at their patients that caused a lot of needless confusion and in many cases led to counter-productive misunderstandings. It could even be in the way a doctor used everyday language in a medical context too casually—a prime example of which I found in my own experience. My surgeons had called my surgery "state of the art." I realized that my family and I thought that meant it was the most advanced—the newest, the best. But during my surgical rotation, I learned that in my case "state of the art" really meant that I was one of the first children to have this procedure.

There were many other opportunities during my medical journey where communication determined the decisions my family made about my care—for better or worse. Lessons learned from these experiences are part of the core curriculum that my partner and dear friend, Val Lantz-Gefroh, and I have created. Our partnership brings together my skills in journalism and my roles as a chronic patient and physician with Val's expertise as a theatre artist resulting in interactive arts and humanities-based training. Our overarching goal is to rewire the way healthcare providers approach communication emphasizing that listening and communicating with our patients is as important as the treatment we deliver. My story reinforces how a simple phrase like "state of the art" can impact the decisions and expectations of a patient and their family. We reflect upon the culture of medicine and the importance of re-examining goals in changing circumstances. In my case, the bag was perceived as a failure because we all were still stuck on goals that were determined with a 15-year-old in mind. When, in fact, there was no failure. I got married, had children, became a journalist and physician educator, and I'm even happy to be "driving a Buick."

We have taught thousands of healthcare providers around the world since first working together 15 years ago on the ground floor of the Alan Alda Center for Communicating Science at Stony Brook University in New York. In 2021, we relocated our efforts to San Diego where we launched the Center for Compassionate Communication at UC San Diego Health's T. Denny Sanford Institute for Empathy and Compassion. Here, we are evaluating the impact of our curriculum on our learners and training health providers to teach this innovative curriculum within their own disciplines through internal and external workshops. Preliminary data not only show an improvement in communication skills but also in their wellness.

Doctors listen when I share that there is more to successful doctoring than diagnosing, treating, prescribing, and operating. My ability to communicate my needs and fears as a patient took on a much deeper dimension when I became a physician and understood firsthand what it was to walk in both my doctor's and patient's shoes. This has not only been vital to my resilience as a permanent patient but also informs my work as an educational leader. I'm not just talking about bedside manner, or even about having the skill and patience to explain complicated things. That's part of it, but just as important is open, two-way communication—encouraging patients to be part of the process, using language they can understand, listening to what they're saying, picking up on what they're feeling. And sometimes having the humility to admit you are human and fallible. People don't like to talk about this, but things happen. Mistakes, sometimes. And sometimes just life.

The most important lesson I have learned throughout my journey is that patients and doctors can learn from one another. I'll never forget the time when I thanked one of my surgeons for my care. He stopped me mid-sentence and said: *No, I should be thanking you for making me a better doctor.*

> Dr. Kaplan-Liss devotes her life's work to the mission of inspiring compassionate communication in medicine. Her research evaluating novel curricula is revealing that arts and humanities based compassionate communication training not only transforms how health providers communicate but also is proving to impact their wellness. In her spare time, she enjoys traveling the world with her family and has a recent addiction to Pilates. Dr. Kaplan-Liss acknowledges Suzy Schultz, journalist extraordinaire who helped her gain perspective and tell her story in writing.

Personal Growth

5

Kathy May Tran, Michael Natter, Elizabeth Roux,
Felippe O. Marcondes, Cassie Craun Ferguson,
Kamal R. Chémali, Perry Pong, and Chi T. Viet

K. M. Tran (✉) · F. O. Marcondes
General Internal Medicine, Department of Medicine, Massachusetts General Hospital, Boston, MA, USA

Department of Medicine, Harvard Medical School, Boston, MA, USA
e-mail: kathy.tran@mgh.harvard.edu

M. Natter
Endocrinology, Diabetes, and Metabolism, Department of Medicine, New York University Langone Medical Center, New York, NY, USA

Department of Medicine, New York University Grossman School of Medicine, New York, NY, USA

E. Roux
Harvard Medical School, Boston, MA, USA

C. C. Ferguson
Pediatric Emergency Medicine, Department of Pediatrics, Children's Wisconsin, Milwaukee, WI, USA

Department of Pediatrics, Medical College of Wisconsin, Milwaukee, WI, USA

K. R. Chémali
Department of Neurology, University Hospitals Cleveland Medical Center, Cleveland, OH, USA

Department of Neurology, Case Western Reserve University School of Medicine, Cleveland, OH, USA

P. Pong
Education and Training, Charles B. Wang Community Health Center, New York, NY, USA

Department of Medicine, Weill Cornell Medical College, New York, NY, USA

C. T. Viet
Department of Oral and Maxillofacial Surgery, Loma Linda University Health, Loma Linda, CA, USA

© The Author(s), under exclusive license to Springer Nature Switzerland AG 2024
M. A. Goldstein, K. M. Tran (eds.), *Becoming a Better Physician*,
https://doi.org/10.1007/978-3-031-69413-4_5

Commentary: Anatomy of Burnout

Michael Natter

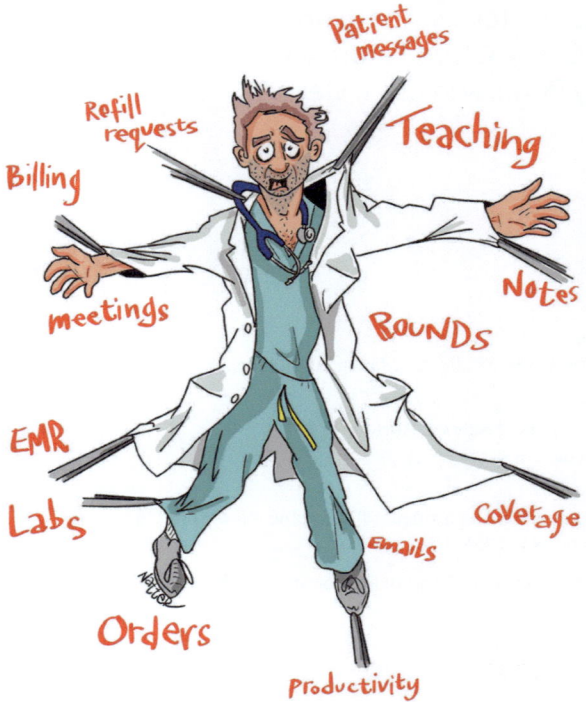

The Blessing of a Bear

Elizabeth Roux

    The sun never sets during Alaskan summers, and I had never felt more alive. A tundra of glacial streams and mountains pierced the sky. Raw, unyielding. No human belonged in this wilderness, and yet we persisted, each trudging step carrying us deeper into humility.
    It was my day to shine, a bright-eyed kid from Florida leading a motley crew across this untamed wilderness. Here there were no vestiges of ocean bliss—moose instead of manatees, permafrost instead of palm trees—but my heart radiated. This

harsh, novel land offered me a most precious gift: a connection to my mother for the first time since cradling her dying frame last year.

I extended my arm, flush from the affection of mosquitos, and pushed through the remaining willows. An iridescent river flowed before me surging with snowmelt. I exhaled with a grin. And then a rustling to my left, a growl reverberating through my spine, and the world lurching to a halt.

A male grizzly bear loomed 20 paces away. Grunting, it reared up on its hind legs and warily sniffed the air. I had never seen a creature so wrathful and magnificent. Shoulder muscles rippled beneath a sheen of mahogany fur. Claws, yellowed and curved like scythes, dangled from its paws. Auburn eyes locked onto mine as the bear slammed down on all fours and broke into a run.

A moment in eternity. I and that enigmatic animal grappled against an indifferent world for the right to carry on unperturbed. With terror hardened by inevitability, I deployed my bear spray directly at its muzzle. A yellow haze erupted and struck the bear square between the eyes before dispersing around me in a cloud of intoxicating agony.

Tears streamed from my eyes and I crumpled to the ground, hefting my backpack on top of me as a final act of salvation. The bear, agitated by the spray but only angrier for it, crashed into me in a torrent of tooth and claw. Its domineering shadow blotted out the sun. Heavy paws forced the breath out of me, and with it my soul.

I feel the lightness of my own existence drifting through the sky. Bereft of fragile body and broken heart, I look down upon a tangible world to see a 16-year-old girl huddled before the mercy of Nature incarnate. Blood oozes from her elbow, head lolling with each thunderous strike from the bear.

Urgency.

Emanating from within my very existence, a dire need to choose: continue drifting toward peace or return to the fervor of the flesh.

I choose peace, and suddenly time transforms into a mere enigma. I live every moment of my life at once, become every version of myself, feel every cruelty and kindness simultaneously in a dazzling cacophony.

I am a newborn on a smoggy Wuhan morning. My birth parents lay me on a street corner near the orphanage and disperse with the haze. Why didn't they leave a note?

I am 11 months old on a plane from Shanghai to Miami. Mom cradles me in her arms as I eat both of our breakfasts and babble to the folks sitting behind us. She and I look nothing alike, but her heart feels like home.

I am 3 years old and giggling as I cling to Mom's back. The water is cold but the sun is warm, and we bob there with the manatees. Mom's eyes sparkle, always the nature lover, and from this moment forevermore I become a nature lover too.

I'm 9 and terrified by the pounding on the front door. It's still dark out. Flashlights, FBI badges, guns. Turns out they are nice men, but here to take Mom's husband away. Mom is distraught and angry, but mostly embarrassed, and also relieved. We had no idea. Good riddance.

I'm 13 and walking barefoot on a beach near our home. White powder sand between my toes. Mom taught me every species of shell that washes up on these shores. An alphabet cone here, a lightning whelk there, a fighting conch with the animal still inside. My hunt continues for her favorite, the apple murex, as a gift for her birthday. A sandpiper skitters over my foot. Salty air.

I'm 15 and playing with my dog. His short black hairs shed relentlessly on our white tile floor, but I couldn't care less. Anything for my buddy. I hear the garage door open; Mom is home. But unlike every other day, she is deflated when she steps into the kitchen. I've never seen her like this before. Eyes pooling with despair, she looks at me and my heart melts. Cancer, she says. We sob through the night.

I'm 16. Chemo has rendered Mom bald and wheelchair-bound. Her nausea comes and goes, her pain always stays, but she still likes to feed the fish and be by the water, so I wheel her out to the dock. She chuckles when a turtle joins the fray. I hope the turtle never leaves.

I'm 16. Angry, terrified, numb. After a month in the hospital, we're back home, but Mom lies in a hospital bed and hospice workers keep buzzing around me. I just want to be alone with her. She hasn't opened her eyes since last night and is sucking in those agonizing breaths. I clutch Mom's hand and tell her that I love her, that I'll be ok. Another shuddering breath.

I'm 16. Mom died 3 days ago. I can't get the memory out of my head of that haunting black body bag, sagging and covered in raindrops, as they carried her down the driveway. The beach is beautiful today and not a soul here. A dolphin jumps near shore, but I feel empty. Nature had always been our thing, and it's just not the same.

I'm 16. Up on stage at my high school auditorium. My teacher nominated me for a scholarship and they're giving it to me. It's not for college, but rather for some sort of adventure out in nature. I choose Alaska—as far from Florida as I can get and as wild as it comes. Plus, Mom and I had always wanted to see a grizzly bear.

Wait. Something is happening.

A warmth envelops me. It is omnipotent and tender and wise and somehow it makes me understand that the peace I chose will not be found here in the sky—not yet, not in this way. I must have faith. My soul once more feels the pull of gravity. Far below the bear strikes again, slashing the backpack in two, and the girl's eyes roll white.

I felt nothing, then everything. A searing pain in my elbow, the weight of the world pressing me into the earth. Another cloud of agony as the others sprang into action deploying more bear spray. The bear bellowed and yielded. My blurry eyes watched its ambling frame disappear over the horizon. I struggled to accept the permanence of its farewell.

Hands feverishly wrapped my elbow in gauze. Mutters of *laceration* and *infection* and *my god it cut her down to the bone*. My eyes drifted from the horizon back to that infinite sky which had welcomed me yet was, for now, unreachable. But I did not mourn. Omnipotence had filled the cracks of my broken heart with faith and hope, joy, and peace. Life brimmed with vitality. All was well.

One decade has passed. Upon returning from Alaska, I found a new family to call my own, graduated from high school, and left the balmy comforts of Florida to study biology at Harvard College. I suffered a concussion, lost my grandmother to stroke, and lost my brother to cancer. I worked and adventured in southern Utah, returned east to Harvard Medical School, and recently got engaged to the love of my life.

There is no definitive arc, theme, or end to this narrative. Life is an ocean whose currents shift unpredictably, and I believe that we ourselves do not change so much as we choose. I choose to dance under the stars, to laugh with the heavens, and to love deeply and fiercely just as much as I permit myself to crawl through depression, stumble through grief, and relive the ravages of the past.

I think often of Alaska, returning to its raw wilderness in my dreams and during my hospital commutes. I see the faces of my birth parents, my mother, my brother, my grandmother, and sometimes even myself as I observe patients and their loved ones. My heart wrenches for their suffering, exalts with their relief, and, outside it all, is wholly fascinated by the human condition. What does it truly mean to live, to die, to love, to lose?

I have come to believe that to live is to love—a love for life and nature, for people and animals—and that losing is a painful yet precious consequence of loving. As for death, it is the end of one journey but perhaps the start of another which our souls, unless untethered to time and tangibility like my brief moment in the sky, cannot yet fathom. I do not presume to have answers, only faith. Faith that stems from that bluebird of a day under a shining Alaskan sun when, with the blessing of a bear, I found grace in the temporary brilliance of life and became free.

> Ms. Roux is a fourth-year medical student at Harvard Medical School and a National Geographic Open Explorer who cares deeply for people, nature, and the exuberant pursuit of life. As a person so too as a budding physician, she hopes to guide others through hardship and healing informed by her background in evolutionary biology and trauma-informed care.

unDOCumented Medicine

Felippe O. Marcondes

I had the dream to go to medical school since I was ten, and I used education as the ultimate proof that I was worthy to be in the United States. I had almost straight As from middle school through college and finished my undergraduate degree *summa cum laude* in three years. By the time I applied to medical school in the fall of 2011, I had a 4.0 GPA. On paper, I attained near academic perfection. Also on paper, I was still undocumented.

December 20, 2012 was one of the happiest days of my life. It was the day I received my only medical school acceptance at the University of Texas Medical Branch in Galveston. I did not know whether to cry or to laugh uncontrollably as I read the much-awaited email. Medical school entering class of 2017. It was a dream come true. After all, I am a DREAMer.

Seven months before, on June 2012, President Barack Obama's executive order, the Deferred Action for Childhood Arrivals (DACA), went into effect. The two-year, renewable, executive action brought to life with a stroke of President Obama's pen was nothing short of a miracle for me. DACA was the main reason I could now attend medical school. And DACA was the only reason I obtained a loan to pay for it. It could not have come at a better time. I became one of the estimated 800,000 DACA recipients in the first year of the program. How many of those young people were going to medical school? Difficult to say. By 2016, I was 1 of 65 undocumented medical students with DACA—nationally.

The academic rigor of medical school was not the heaviest weight I carried. For four years, I felt like I shouldered the weight of 11 million undocumented immigrants who I was representing. In addition to learning the cranial nerves, the nuances of pharmacology, and the art and science of medicine, I also remembered. I remembered where I came from and what being a medical student meant for my parents. I felt so much pride to represent and experience something my parents could not. I wanted to give them back a bit of the pride that being undocumented had stripped them of. But no matter how well I performed in medical school, there were things I could not make better for my parents. Giving them health insurance was one of them.

At school, I learned the importance of colon and breast cancer screening. But trying to get my own parents to go in for a colonoscopy felt like preaching down. I knew they were uninsured. I was uninsured. And neither of us could afford the $3000-dollar out-of-pocket cost for a colonoscopy. In Brazil, there is a saying that "a household saint cannot perform any miracles." That was me: Saint Felippe, the doctor-in-training who could not save his own household from uninsurance. That was hard for me to accept. It still is.

The feeling of powerlessness from knowing to being able to do was not restricted to my parents. I experienced it with my own patients. Treating undocumented patients as an undocumented medical student, and later internal medicine resident, was especially difficult in Texas. Aside from occasionally functioning as an ad hoc Spanish interpreter, most of the time I felt powerless. Not because I lacked medical knowledge. I knew that would come with time. But because of the moral injury of preventable suffering that I witnessed. One particular case stays with me to this day. I met Mr. P, a 65-year-old man with end-stage renal disease (ESRD) and diabetes who was admitted almost every month through the emergency department for "compassionate" hemodialysis for hyperkalemia or uremic symptoms. The whole experience was all but compassionate. One of estimated 5500 to 8857 undocumented immigrants with ESRD in the United States, Mr. P did not speak English. He was uninsured and undocumented. Like me. Behind California, Texas has the second-largest population of undocumented immigrants in the United States. However, unlike California—which offers standard-of-care hemodialysis three times a week—Texas offers predominantly emergency-only hemodialysis to undocumented immigrants. He did not have regular outpatient follow-up because he could not afford it. He could not receive a transplant either. That day, he was dialyzed and discharged home. My heart sank as I thought despite my best intentions, the healthcare system placed barriers that made it nearly impossible for him to receive the care he needed. On self-assessment, my diagnosis was clear: moral distress. And medical school and residency did not prepare me to treat that.

In an important way, my undocumented status helps me to be a better doctor for my patients. Having faced language barriers when seeking healthcare to settling medical debt with collections due to inability to afford healthcare, I empathize. I deeply empathize with my disadvantaged patients and their struggles to have access to a primary care physician, their difficulty paying for their medications, and their struggles to be seen by a healthcare system that was designed to favor privilege. They often feel invisible. Being undocumented can feel invisible. I am their primary care doctor. And my life experiences help me see their pain. Even if it is for 15 or 30 minutes at a time.

Eleven years ago, going to medical school seemed impossible because I didn't have "papers." Today, the diploma paper on my wall reads, "Felippe Ottoni Marcondes, M.D." I am a doctor. Albeit an undocumented to one. Yet, I still try to achieve my way out of the feelings of never belonging, of living in immigration limbo. DACA is limbo. I thought being in a place of academic and medical excellence would quiet down my thoughts of inadequacy.

I am now a physician-researcher at the Massachusetts General Hospital and Harvard Medical School. Once I got to Harvard—the pinnacle of my medical and academic career aspiration—my mindset needed to change. To continue to achieve my way out of my insecurities centered on my immigration status was not sustainable. A slow—and at times painful—process started of letting go of the need to continuously prove I deserve to be here, in the United States and at Harvard. I am starting to realize I do not have to prove myself. I need to *be* myself. My full Latino, undocumented, doctor self.

> Dr. Marcondes is a primary care physician who is an advocate for undocumented immigrants, quality healthcare for all, and lifestyle medicine in patient care. He is the proud husband, son, and brother of immigrants. A version of this essay by Dr. Marcondes appeared as a Graphic Perspective in the *New England Journal of Medicine*.

Overcoming Overwhelm

Cassie Craun Ferguson

I am a pediatric emergency medicine physician. I care for kids with colds, Strep throat, appendicitis, and gunshot wounds. More and more, I also care for kids with "behavioral health problems," a lackluster umbrella term for kids who are depressed, anxious, or dangerous to themselves or others.

One evening, I was caring for a 7-year-old child with autism in Room 7 whose behavior at home had become so violent and disruptive that his adoptive parents feared he might hurt himself or his younger sister. My plan was to ask our social worker to provide his mom with a list of resources for respite care. However, as they waited, the child became increasingly anxious and distressed. He began pacing around the room, pulling equipment off the walls, pushing away the nurse's attempts to help him back into bed. His mom, previously calm, had begun crying and then began screaming loudly enough for the entire 22-bed department to hear,

> WHY WON'T ANYONE HELP US?
> NO ONE EVER LISTENS TO ME!
> I CAN'T DO THIS ANYMORE!

I stood outside of their room in the hallway, watching it all happen from a distance. I hesitated briefly but then walked toward the room, slid the heavy glass doors open, and went in. I knew then that there was a time in the not-so-distant past when I would have slunk back to my computer and waited for our social worker to come and speak with her, a time when this mother's suffering would have frightened and overwhelmed me. Even remembering this now, I feel a pang of shame admitting that, but sharing stories like this is about telling the truth.

To understand what changed, we have to rewind 3 years to March 2020 when COVID-19 shut the world down. My kids' schools had just closed, we were donning hazmat suits and respirators at work, and my husband was furloughed from work. The world was upside down.

Luckily, having lived my whole life with an unshakeable premonition of disaster, I was ready for a pandemic. Within a week of the shutdown, I had an aggressively detailed plan. My kids would learn math on Khan Academy and creative writing from *The New York Times*. I would work in the ED in the evenings and on weekends, when my husband could be home with the kids. I would write all the manuscripts I had intended to write over the past decade, create engaging, interactive online classes for my medical students, sanitize our groceries, do yoga at lunchtime, and meditate before bed.

As the weeks went by, each of my plans broke apart. I moved frenetically between appearing engaged on work Zoom calls, pleading with my 6-year-old to get off the floor and do writer's workshop, and Googling "how to tell if my teenager is depressed." I collected N95s and homemade masks from neighbors, fielded phone calls from medical students whose family members were dying from COVID, and unconvincingly reassured colleagues that *we would be okay*. Like a shark, constant movement became the only thing keeping me alive.

Until May, that is, when my body began its surrender to the whirling catastrophe my mind had become.

It started with early morning awakenings. Then unrelenting headaches. Food started to taste unnecessary and bland. I forgot meetings and appointments, left work unfinished, was disengaged from my husband, family, and friends. Before shifts in the ED, I would sit in my car, immobile and breathless, my legs heavy and unwilling to carry my body inside the war zone our hospital had become. By the end of May, I was having trouble remembering to shower. When the people around me offered to help, I would stare at them blankly, lacking the insight to ask for what I needed and utterly bereft of hope to believe things could be different.

In her book *The Age of Overwhelm*, author Laura van Dernoot Lipsky points out that one of the self-constructed barriers to managing overwhelm is our endorsement of the notion that "being who we are and not being overwhelmed are mutually exclusive." By the time the pandemic rolled around, I had been operating under this premise for nearly three decades: Believing that the seat of privilege I occupied meant I was to assume the obligation of taking on more and more. Believing that what needed fixing could be fixed. Becoming indignant when I was told it couldn't be. Always anticipating what would be next to go wrong. Always in dress rehearsal for the next tragedy. I was firmly attached to the view of myself as someone who would *proudly* never get to the bottom of her to-do list.

But in May 2020, this way of taking on the world finally broke me apart. Navigating a pandemic as a physician and a mom had exploded the background hum of anxiety I typically tolerated, and layered over that was the shame I felt for falling short of how I believed I was supposed to be serving my patients, my family, my students, and my community.

A good friend gently pushed me to speak to my doctor, who prescribed an antidepressant. My sleep returned, and my headaches stopped. This was lifesaving.

With the ground beneath me again, I began to piece my life back together intentionally, knowing I couldn't go back to living in a state of chronic overwhelm. The tools on offer for overcoming overwhelm, however—bullet journals, to-do list apps, self-checkout kiosks, DIY coffee enema kits—were insulting (albeit alluringly accessible) and deviously designed to take advantage of those of us who spend too much time on Instagram and have, as my therapist would say, "unrelenting standards."

What I really wanted that these tools could not help me with—although, to be honest, I haven't tried the coffee enema—was to stop yelling at my kids when I couldn't find my car keys. I wanted to feel capable again. I wanted to see my patients as whole humans with more to offer than the problems they brought me to solve. More than anything, I wanted to be *satisfied with the present moment,* whatever it contained.

And in the last three years, with help from medication, therapy, hours of podcasts, and a bookshelf that looks like the self-help section of a Barnes and Noble, I have learned that these things are possible. *Sometimes.*

They are possible when I engage in rituals that give me a sense of stability. When I sit in my living room before everyone in the house wakes up and close my eyes and count my breaths until the sun rises.

They are possible when I am in community with friends or colleagues—the people who know me in detail, who tell me the truth about their lives, and show up when I tell them not to.

They are possible when I am content with just doing the next right thing, and when I loosen my grip on the urge to fix it all (and the privileged delusion that I could).

But the most revolutionary practice I implemented in the past three years is self-compassion. Even when I sleep in, or disappoint a good friend, or am called to care for a patient with problems I cannot solve, I extend myself the same compassion, grace, and mercy that I would naturally extend to others when they fall short or feel as if they are failing. Dr. Kristen Neff and Dr. Christopher Germer, psychologists who study self-compassion, describe it as having three components: (1) speaking to yourself kindly, as you would a good friend; (2) recognizing the universality of our difficult experiences; and (3) being willing to observe our negative thoughts with curiosity and clarity.

I admit it was awkward at first—I have spent most of my life believing the worst of myself—but with practice, having compassion for myself has changed how I walk through the world, how I parent, how I teach, and how I care for patients.

Which brings us back to the child and his mother in Room 7.

Sliding open the glass doors, I walked into the room and sat cross-legged next to the patient's mother on the ground who was so distraught she didn't seem to notice that I had come into the room. As she screamed, I purposefully noticed my breath coming in, and imagined I was flooding my body with compassion. As she cried out for help, I noticed my breath going out, imagining I was flooding her with compassion. Then simply, breathing in, I said to myself "One for me," and breathing out, "One for you." Her screaming stopped. I gently put my hand on her knee and we sat together, briefly suspended in the care that arises from 360° of compassionate presence.

> Dr. Ferguson is a mom to three boys—Ben, Will, and Nick—and wife of a radiologist named Brad whom she met at the Medical College of Wisconsin as a medical student. She is also an attending physician in the emergency department at Children's Wisconsin and the director for both the *Good Doctor* well-being thread and the *Health Systems Science* thread at the Medical College of Wisconsin School of Medicine in Milwaukee. Informally, she is referred to by her colleagues as the "Chief Feelings Officer" which reveals her interests in fostering well-being, connecting to the joy inherent in medicine, and destigmatizing mental health seeking among medical students, trainees, and practicing physicians.

The Frustration of a Musician-Turned-Physician

Kamal R. Chémali

"Son, do you want to live as an exile, or do you want to live and work in your own country?" I was expressing my ambitious plans to go to Paris to study to become a concert pianist when my father posed this question. Without hesitation, my answer came naturally and resolutely: "No! I want to live in my country!" My father's response was equally spontaneous and direct: "Then choose another profession." And so, I embarked on my next best option: medicine.

If given the chance, I would make the same decision again. However, a lingering sense of frustration and regret remains deep within me. Even now, after attending awe-inspiring concerts or listening to magnificent recordings, I can't help but entertain the grandiose notion that I could have become the pianist of my dreams. Alas, these lofty thoughts are swiftly replaced by the harsh reality of everyday life.

Lebanon is a country ravaged by consecutive wars, with only a brief period of peace and prosperity following World War II. The French mandate, which lasted from the end of World War I until the country's independence in 1943, contributed to a remarkable cultural development and durable tradition. This was a stark contrast to the oppressive rule of the Ottoman Empire that had kept the country in a state of obscurity for over 500 years. Like many children of my generation, I began piano lessons at the age of 7. However, the Lebanese "Civil War," which broke out when I was just 8 years old and persisted until shortly before my 24th birthday, casted a tragic shadow over my musical future.

My teacher saw potential in me from a young age, referring to me as "a talented child." I developed a love for classical music when I was just 3 or 4 years old, thanks to my father's modest LP collection. It mainly consisted of Beethoven's nine symphonies, the Deutsche Gramophone 1963 recording by the Berlin Philharmonic conducted by Karajan, and Mozart's 40th and 41st symphonies under the direction of Karl Böhm, with 2 of Bach's 4 orchestral suites. These captivating compositions became the soundtrack of my childhood, played on either my small turntable or my father's larger one. By the time I turned 5, I could sing along to all the melodies when asked. However, while I had natural ability, learning piano seriously proved to be a different challenge altogether. I began with great excitement, but as I faced more difficult pieces, my enthusiasm waned. My parents joked, "You were eager to become the next Beethoven, but now that you realize the hard work involved, you're ready to quit!" To keep me engaged without overwhelming me, they asked my teacher to reduce the amount of practice. Indeed, I regained interest and even started to compose at the age of 10.

Through the instability, my teacher believed in me and encouraged me to pursue a more serious musical education at the prestigious National Conservatory of Music. With his guidance, I prepared and successfully gained admission. I was filled with immense joy. However, on the very first day, tragedy struck. A car bomb exploded in front of the conservatory, obliterating the building, causing death and injuries. I narrowly escaped with my life. I couldn't bring myself to touch or even look at a piano for nearly a year afterward, consumed by grief tainted by the senseless violence.

I still held onto the aspiration of becoming a pianist. Over the following years, I doubled my practice time and studied music theory, harmony, and counterpoint—mostly on my own but following the curriculum of the National Conservatory. My childhood teacher guided me, transforming from a despised figure into a cherished friend.

During my college years, I had already made a conscious and practical decision to pursue a degree in biology as a pre-medical student. At the same time, my skills as a pianist flourished. I explored improvisation and delved into genres beyond classical music. I directed church choirs and a university chamber orchestra, and I even formed a band at my university in which I served as a keyboardist and vocalist.

Before my medical journey began, I penned a poetic vow to my "True Love"—music. Eventually and gradually, that vow was tested as medicine took center stage in my life. I grappled with the frustration of a scarce rendezvous with my beloved piano. The irresistible urge to play whenever I stumbled upon a piano left me yearning for purpose.

To give direction to my musical aimlessness, I hatched a plan: play music for hospitalized patients. Initially, I justified my personal need to play more piano with the assumption that music might be healing to my patients. Little did I know, there was already a trove of scientific literature supporting the profound effects of music on health, to expedite healing and decrease hospital stays. My intuition was right! In a war-torn country where access to medical literature was scarce, I genuinely and mistakenly thought I was the sole medical student bringing the healing power of music to patients.

My medical path brought me to the United States for a neurology residency at Case Western Reserve University, in a city renowned for its vibrant music scene. My move to Cleveland, Ohio was driven by two major dreams: finding an inspiring role model in medicine and seeking a remarkable piano teacher. I yearned for an Albert Schweitzer-like figure to admire. During residency, with the advent of the internet, I pored over medical literature and was astounded by the multitude of studies affirming the therapeutic power of music, particularly in the realm of neurological diseases. It even crossed my mind that my choice of neurology as a specialty was driven by a desire to understand the profound impact of music on the brain.

Yet still, I questioned my identity and purpose. The relentless inner struggle made each day a battleground of choices. Every morning, I contemplated abandoning medicine in favor of music, only to change my mind by evening. In my darkest moments, I also considered giving up music, my first calling, the thing that flowed through my veins, echoed in my soul. I let my piano gather dust for months, thinking that avoiding it might bring closure and peace. But I could not bear to lose my true love and eventually I would return to my instrument, embracing it as a lifeline.

With time, I accepted that music would always be a part of my life, albeit a smaller role. I found balance with the realization that the piano didn't require all my time, just a few dedicated hours a week to practice. My world became "livable" again, as I found a certain harmony between my two passions.

That livability developed because of a decisive step to embrace both worlds simultaneously—at least the intersection of them. The world of music and medicine was far from easy. This intersection was relatively uncharted territory compared to the long-established traditions of each. It was a domain that lacked definition and recognition unless one pursued music therapy as a specialized field. Let it be known that a musician-doctor is not synonymous with a music therapist. The latter requires a specific curriculum that encompasses more than musical listening or performance—a bachelor's, master's, or even doctorate. That distinction left me exasperated. I felt compelled to pursue both music and medicine, but I no longer identified as a musician, nor was I a music therapist.

With an open mind, I immersed myself in the world of music therapists and professional musicians, drawing inspiration from each expertise. With their guidance and collaboration, I researched and discovered the profound impact of music on the human brain and on neurological diseases. I eagerly integrated music into my clinical encounters. Music became a valuable tool, a unique instrument that enabled me to grasp and even modulate patients' emotions. Armed with prior musical studies and a solid understanding of music theory, I unraveled the intricate components of melody, rhythm, harmony, and tempo to create playlists tailored to the unique needs of each patient.

Today, I continue to collaborate with musicians, composers, music therapists, and other musician-physicians to explore the intersection of music and medicine. We research the therapeutic applications of music for patients in various medical settings, and we advocate for the integration of music into healthcare systems so that more patients can benefit. Music has become an integral part of my identity as a neurologist, and it provides a means to express and connect with patients on a profound level. However, I confess that there are still moments when frustration resurfaces. The lingering sense of regret and dissatisfaction sometimes weighs heavily on my mind. I work actively to navigate and reconcile these mixed emotions. I remind myself that both music and medicine offer a unique perspective on patients, and each enhances the care I give to patients. Life does not always go as planned and there is a lot of irony. I did not pursue music as a professional because I wanted to live in my home country, so I pursued medicine instead. Now that I am a physician, I live as an expatriate. And, I did pursue music after all, in a different and unexpected way, an alternative path of purpose, joy, and fulfillment.

> Dr. Chémali is an academic neurologist specializing in autonomic medicine and neuromuscular neurology. Before becoming a doctor, he was a conservatory-trained pianist who was dreaming of the concert stages of the world. Instead, he brought together his passion and his work into the field of music and medicine. He is a firm believer in the transformative power of music in health and disease and uses it in practicing neurology.

Are you Chinese? Yes, and I'm Asian American Too

Perry Pong

Every day for the last 17 years, I have cared for the mostly Chinese diaspora of New York City. When I look into their faces, I see myself. When I discuss their struggles, I see my own challenges. When I hear their dreams, I see those of my own family.

My mother was born in China. Her own mother had passed away in childbirth. She came as a war bride at the tender age of 16, though it stated 18 on her papers—the first of her family to come to the United States. San Francisco's Chinatown was her village, and she made friends in the sewing factory with whom she could share her experiences. My father was a generation ahead, born in Fort Worth, Texas. His own father died young, leaving my father to care for three younger brothers. He was fortunate to get a job in the United States Post Office. An old photo shows him to be 1 of 2 Chinese out of 50 employees at his site. Luckily, since I was the youngest child, I had nice hand-me-downs from my cousins, like my treasured book *The Big Snow*, which I read every night before bed. I also had enough change to buy candy bars at the corner grocery.

Those candy bars led to innumerable cavities, which led to trips to one of the only dentists in Chinatown. I still recoil when I think about the sounds of the drill. Mom would dutifully take me and pay cash. His waiting room overflowed, and I'm sure he was only popular because we had nowhere else to go. My pediatrician was an affable Chinese American man, a proud University of California Berkeley and Creighton Medical School graduate, who often injected me with penicillin whenever my mom took me in for a fever. "Miracle medicine," my mother insisted with conviction.

My parents passed their Chinese values to their children. The immigrant drive for economic security and, by extension, educational achievement for the next generation, were instilled in me since early childhood. These values were an undercurrent that propelled me along a flowing river, pervading everything that I did. Study and do well. Respect your elders. My mother's relatives and friends were pleased. "He's so good. He's so obedient and quiet." As long as you excelled in school, you would be recognized. It didn't matter what your parents did for a living. In a way, I was recognized, but my elementary-school teachers and college professors still called me "smart and quiet." Fair or unfair, that is a common label given to many Asians and Asian Americans.

As I journeyed through college, medical school, and residency, I kept on that path. Study hard, master the material, and get the grades. Follow the rules, keep your head down, and don't stick out. Sure, this was more than adequate in high school, functional in college, and acceptable in medical school. However, this upbringing, as a logical consequence, led to more passive than active learning.

I started to come to the realization after medical school that I could only excel so far obliging the tenets of my parents. As an Asian, I might memorize volumes precisely and accurately. This was indeed valuable. As an Asian American, I might ask the key question, "Why?" This was also just as important. Why does asthma manifest this way? Why is it important to use steroids? The bells of connections and understanding went off in my brain. In residency, my questions continued. Why are we ordering this test? Why are we choosing this treatment? If I embraced both parts of who I am, I could be more, do more.

Being Asian American didn't mean that I had to shed my Chinese upbringing. On the contrary, embracing my Asian American identity could help my Chinese identity grow and become greater. Question authority, learn for yourself, and make an independent analysis based on evidence and critical thinking. With these strategies, an Asian American physician could give the best care to patients.

As I began caring for the Chinese immigrant diaspora and other Asian Americans, I kept asking questions. Not only do I ask, "What do you do for work?" but also I ask, "How many days and hours do you work?" Often the answer is six days a week. Not only do I ask, "Where do you live?" but also I ask, "Who lives at home?" Sometimes I learn that the patient, mom, dad, grandparents, and two siblings all live in a two-bedroom apartment. Not only do I ask, "How many children do you have?" but also I ask, "What are they doing now?" Only then do I discover and normalize feelings of disconnection as their children adopt a language and behaviors that are foreign to them. Teenagers who stretch their wings and extend their boundaries are often seen as rejecting their Chinese upbringing and disrespecting their elders, instead of evolving on a normal social progression. I realize that theirs is a similar to my own progression in my medical journey. As a trusted physician, I can help my patients understand how their kids are Asian American. We can even laugh about it.

My health center, staffed by majority first-generation Chinese Americans, has been awarded a gold-medal designation for diabetes care for several years in a row. I am proud of our health center, staff, and patients. Our attention to detail and care for each patient are excellent. I foresee, however, that even in our diligent endeavors we will plateau, as if we are nearing the bend of the hemoglobin dissociation curve, unless we are also able to grow beyond the old values.

Supervisors are appointed to direct, and also, they should be checked—by frontline staff, nurses, mid-levels, and physicians alike. Rules are made to be followed, and also, they should be questioned and even broken as needed. Strategies are developed to guide practice, and also, they should be reassessed. Purposeful and creative decision-making by all role groups and levels is necessary. We cannot stifle an individual's growth and development or leave out their collective experience; in fact, these things should be encouraged. Staff who say, "You're in charge. You tell us what to do," will often be the ones to later say, "Administration doesn't listen to us. They order us around." We need to empower these staff to speak up, stand up, so that they can be active and involved in processes and procedures. If we set their spirit free, they and our organization will be healthier and better. It may take another generation or two, but I believe it will happen.

I am Chinese. I am Asian American. I benefit from the immigrant experience because I am humble and grateful for where I came from. Appreciation of both experiences propels me to strive higher and gives me hope, to excel at what I do and to help my patients and community. In the next generation, I foresee that Asian Americans will foster even more openness, inquiry, and value in the organizations that service the Chinese diaspora. And we will remain just as respectful to and appreciative of our Chinese roots.

> Dr. Pong has dedicated his career to fostering work cultures whereby all patients walking in the door feel they are cared for and respected. He enjoys teaching the next generation to find joy and wonder in primary care.

Embracing Loss to Find Fulfillment

Chi T. Viet

"When you told me we were going to be lifelong friends, I didn't think it would be this short." I was seated by her bedside in the last days of her life. Our difficult conversation, centered around how to set her up to be discharged home to die, was made even more difficult because speaking had become too painful, leaving her to communicate only by writing. I looked at the sentence she had jotted, speechless.

Just one year before, I had diagnosed the tongue cancer that would kill her. She was a young woman who had never smoked, the type of patient whose cancer acts in a disturbingly aggressive manner, leaving us completely blindsided. I had removed the majority of her tongue, lymph nodes in the neck, and performed extensive tongue reconstruction. She then underwent a difficult course of chemotherapy and radiation. The treatments robbed her of the ability to speak and eat, left her with chronic pain and dependence on both opioids and a feeding tube. But the cancer came back with a vengeance, this time widely metastatic.

When she had entrusted me to be her cancer surgeon, I had promised her that I would see her frequently for the rest of her life. It is a declaration I make to all patients at their initial office consultation, with the hope that they will actually be in the minority who survive the diagnosis of oral cancer and that we will be lifelong partners in their treatment journey. But it is also in these same office walls where I discuss hospice when their cancer is no longer curable, preparing them and their family for their death at home, especially if a carotid blowout is imminent. Through the years I have said goodbye to most of my cancer patients with this difficult discussion. And although I have gained experience as a surgeon, coping with the loss of my patients has only become harder, especially since I could not help but feel responsible for their outcome.

Loss permeates my career and my life. As I spoke to my patient and she wrote to me, I thought about an earlier loss that led me to become a cancer surgeon and scientist in the first place. I was meant to be a general dentist, the daughter of two dentists who had grown up in their dental clinic. As a first-year dental student doing research on oral cancer, one patient I enrolled was a Vietnamese immigrant who had just come to the United States with his wife and four children. He was diagnosed with late-stage tongue cancer that had become incurable. I volunteered as his Vietnamese language interpreter. During his visits, I saw the fear of loss in his eyes. He only had months to survive the all-consuming disease before leaving his wife and young children in a foreign country. He is the reason I shifted my entire career trajectory. In addition to dental school, I enrolled in a PhD program focused on cancer research, then completed medical school, oral maxillofacial surgery residency, and a head and neck cancer ablation and microvascular reconstruction fellowship—decisions that followed naturally when I made it my life's purpose to help cancer patients live longer, better quality lives through thoughtful research and surgery. By all measures, my training path led me to a successful academic career as a surgeon scientist. Yet peeling back the accomplishments, what is left is the feeling of guilt and a heightened sense of hopelessness, knowing that my best efforts would never be enough as my patients are still dying.

The training brought a different kind of loss into my life—personal sacrifice that I did not foresee. For my entire 20s and much of my 30s, I lived apart from family, missed holidays and celebrations. When my husband and I were married and when I gave birth to our daughter, I could only spare a week before returning to residency. I still wonder what it would be like to be a mother who could spend a full maternity leave to bond with her daughter. The first time she crawled or walked was in a daycare, while I was in fellowship training. And more recently as an attending surgeon, my path to give my daughter a sibling has been wrought with struggles—infertility issues that too many women physicians have an intimate understanding of. As physicians, we are trained to be masters of self-sacrifice and to rationalize our pain as being necessary for our career, to the point where we can become self-destructive. If we are fortunate, we do not also destroy our relationships in the process. My relationship with my family, husband, and friends saw its darkest moments while I was in training. I am grateful, however, that they offered love and empathy, even when I was too worn down to reciprocate.

I have struggled to cope with the loss and hopelessness that bled into every aspect of my life as a cancer surgeon. At first, I ignored this pain out of self-preservation, thinking that I could prevent my own suffering. With more life experience, I realized that my suffering came from expecting things to be permanent when they are not. Loss is a part of living. Once I embraced the impermanence of life and the pain of my own losses, I was able to focus intently on the present moment. I started gardening as a form of meditation after I became an attending surgeon, allowing me to come home to my thoughts in the present. One orchid gifted by a patient has turned into hundreds, now treasured in a greenhouse I built in my backyard. Many of these orchids have outlived the people who gifted them. I learned to integrate my work and home life, to intertwine them rather than compartmentalize them—bringing my daughter to my clinic and research lab and sharing freely with my husband the grief I feel in my work.

Now that I have discovered how to embrace the pain of loss and to know that it is the past, I am reminded about how wonderful it is to breathe freely in the present, when many of my patients cannot breathe without feeling pain. And with that I have found true fulfillment in my work and life.

> Dr. Viet is a surgeon scientist with a clinical practice and research lab focused on improving outcomes in patients with head and neck cancer. She enjoys cooking for her husband and daughter, spending time in her garden, and mentoring the next generation of thoughtful surgeons and scientists.

Love and Loss

6

Michael Jellinek, Kerri Palamara McGrath,
Imani E. McElroy, Mark Allan Goldstein, Maria Trent,
Clara Baselga-Garriga, and Gleeson Rebello

M. Jellinek
Child Psychiatry Service, Department of Psychiatry, Massachusetts General Hospital, Boston, MA, USA

Department of Psychiatry, Harvard Medical School, Boston, MA, USA

K. P. McGrath
General Internal Medicine, Department of Medicine, Massachusetts General Hospital, Boston, MA, USA

Department of Medicine, Harvard Medical School, Boston, MA, USA

I. E. McElroy
General Surgery Residency Program, Massachusetts General Hospital, Boston, MA, USA

M. A. Goldstein (✉)
Adolescent and Young Adult Medicine, Department of Pediatrics, Massachusetts General Hospital, Boston, MA, USA

Department of Pediatrics, Harvard Medical School, Boston, MA, USA
e-mail: mgoldstein@mgh.harvard.edu

M. Trent
Adolescent and Young Adult Medicine, Johns Hopkins Children's Center, Baltimore, MD, USA

Department of Pediatrics, Johns Hopkins Medicine, Baltimore, MD, USA

C. Baselga-Garriga
Harvard Medical School, Boston, MA, USA

G. Rebello
Pediatric Orthopedic Surgery, Department of Orthopedics, Mass General Brigham, Boston, MA, USA

Department of Orthopaedic Surgery, Harvard Medical School, Boston, MA, USA

© The Author(s), under exclusive license to Springer Nature Switzerland AG 2024
M. A. Goldstein, K. M. Tran (eds.), *Becoming a Better Physician*,
https://doi.org/10.1007/978-3-031-69413-4_6

Commentary: Abe

Michael Jellinek

> Doubting his future
> Anxious and depressed every day,
> More so every night
> Feeling undeserving of gift or lover
>
> Apple geek, artist, philosopher
> Writer, entrepreneur, investor
> Comic and mentor
> Ragged shoes amidst plenty
>
> Searching, remembering everything
> Kant to Seinfeld
> Needing six gloves
> To sometimes find two
>
> Brilliant and funny
> Loved but guarded.
> Angry, yet most often kind
> Distant but often present
>
> Dreading his longevity
> Panicky, desperate for sleep
> Misjudging his illicit relief
> He never awoke…and is missed every day.

> Dr. Jellinek is a child psychiatrist who continues to see patients, consult, and teach.

The Gifts Grief Brings: One Physician's Journey Through Grief After Loss

Kerri Palamara McGrath

I was not worried about being a good doctor to my primary care patients. I cared about my patients, listened to them, did my best for them, and had wonderful relationships with many of them. As a more than full-time working mom to two young kids, I had a busy, chaotic lifestyle, but it all seemed to work. I was the panelist on all the parenting panels discussing how to build a career while still being present with your family. I wasn't looking to evolve or transform into a better version of myself. I was content with my professional and personal lives.

And then, one day, my world was changed forever. I got the call that no parent wanted to receive—my nanny screaming into the phone about an accident, an emergency medical services official asking me how soon I could get to the local hospital and if I had someone to drive me. I begged them to take the kids to Mass General, where I was working, but they told me they had to go to the closest hospital. I should have known then that something terrible was happening. I drove myself across town, frantically trying to find my way through traffic while gathering information on what might have happened to my children while also trying to contact my husband who was on the other side of the country on business.

My husband, Brendan, asked me if he should go to the airport, and I didn't know what to tell him. I called my nanny again, and an ER doctor answered. He told me to try to stay calm and focus on driving, and that he would tell me more when I arrived. I told him I knew what he was doing and asked him to tell me the bad news, he said, "If you know what I am doing, then you know why I am doing it. I will meet you at the entrance. Pull right up and give your keys to the officer standing next to me." By then, I knew someone was dead.

I got there in a panic, to find the ER staff doing a slow code on my almost 3-year-old son, Colin. Our 4-year-old daughter was nowhere to be found, but I heard someone tell me she was going to live. I looked at the attending, who said, "I understand you are a physician. We have been coding your son for 20 minutes. His pupils are dilated and there is no pulse." I begged her to stop and to let me hold him. After gently placing Colin in my arms, all but a few left the room. As if, by magic, our family priest suddenly arrived in the ER bay to give him last rights and help me find my daughter.

I called Brendan, who was driving to the airport, and told him to pull over. I didn't make him wait any longer. It was all over the news. Our son was dead, and our daughter needed several surgeries. We cried together as I held Colin in my arms and cradled the phone against my ear. I don't remember how I hung up the phone because I would not let Colin go. At that moment, I thought our world was never going to be the same. I didn't know then how I would ever get up from that chair, let alone go on with raising our wounded daughter.

I remember the day we left the hospital without Colin as if it were yesterday. Leaving the hospital without your child goes against everything that feels right or normal. It went against my parental instinct to care for and protect my child. My body and mind wanted to fight it, yet there was no way to win. We wondered how we could go home without him, and how we would ever get through losing him. This wasn't what our story was supposed to be, and now we were stuck with this life of sadness. I remember feeling as if we received a life sentence of pain, forced to live the rest of our lives without our son, which felt like an eternity. I wanted to scream out, "I had a son!" as if I needed to remind the world and myself that he lived—that he existed.

Many say there is no loss greater than the loss of a child. In the beginning, our grief felt as if it was everywhere, and it was out of our control. People told us over time, we'd cry less, feel less pain, and begin to have some control over when and where we cried, and how we felt our grief. I found it hard to believe, especially when I would see reminders of my son everywhere. When I would walk into a store, I might need to walk out because there was a little boy and his mom shopping. But, eventually, the pain lessened. Eventually I was able to feel something other than grief.

I felt as if I would never be able to go back to work. Being a physician had always been part of my identity, and now it felt meaningless—my identity was as a grieving mother. That was all I could see and feel. After about 9 months, I slowly returned to seeing patients. We were careful about whom I would see, how many patients were in my schedule, and what they were told before seeing me (rather than ask Dr. Palamara how she is doing, simply say, "It's great to see you back.") Despite that, it still didn't feel right. I still felt lost in the shadow of the person, physician, and mother I used to be. I struggled to feel empathy at times and to connect with patients in the way I used to. I couldn't let them in, nor did I have the emotional bandwidth to be let into their suffering or struggles as I had in the past. I decided it wasn't working, and I couldn't continue this way. I sat with a dear physician friend who herself had experienced loss, and together, we hatched a Plan B. I would approach my division chief, tell him I couldn't be a primary care physician anymore, and change to urgent care. For the first time in months, it felt like maybe I could still be a doctor even with the gaping hole inside of me. Then the COVID-19 pandemic began.

Experts in posttraumatic growth encourage you to find the gift that your loss brings you. Some call it the blessings or the silver linings. I struggled with this enormously in the wake of Colin's death. How could losing my son be a blessing? How could there be any silver lining (note—I still dislike that term despite finding acceptance years later)? Despite my resistance, the COVID-19 pandemic brought me three perspective-changing gifts that I have come to appreciate.

The first gift was that my skills as a physician and leader were REALLY needed, but in new ways. I didn't have to be a primary care doctor in my practice—in fact, I couldn't be one. But I could be a physician in the testing tents and help run the respiratory illness clinic and the field hospital. I threw myself into all the COVID-19-related work that I could get my hands on, as an escape and to feel good about being a doctor again—to find a new physician identity for myself.

The second gift was that when I was asked, "How are you doing?" the assumption was no longer about how my grief was, which I often didn't want to answer, but rather how was I coping with the pandemic. It was a relief to return to conversational norms.

And finally, the third gift was that I no longer had the market cornered on grief. It was everywhere. And I had eyes that could see it in ways that few others could visualize. It did more than restore my empathy and ability to connect—it supercharged it. I suddenly had a new expertise in grief, coping, and resilience that few others had the language for, and it presented ways to be helpful to others that has forever changed who I am as a physician and colleague.

Sitting with someone's grief and not trying to take it away or change it is a skill that few possess. Listening without trying to fix is something many people spend a lifetime trying to learn. I had spent the prior 18 months surrounded by grief, in therapy, supporting my family and myself, and learning how to survive despite our loss and trauma. I had learned and was living these skills every day. Suddenly, I could hear and see patients differently as they faced the challenges that the pandemic brought to them. As they experienced loss and stress, I could help them name their struggle and their emotions and help them feel seen and heard. I was a different physician now: one that was not afraid of other's deep and dark emotions; one that could sit and hold them for others; and one that could realize that sometimes listening is the real medicine, rather than whatever drug I might prescribe or advice I might offer. That authenticity reinvigorated my sense of purpose and meaning at a time when many had lost theirs. It was, in fact, a gift that my loss and the pandemic gave me and for which I was grateful.

This is my journey of posttraumatic growth—of surviving my worst nightmare and learning how to live again, in a way that I was changed for the better. My loss did not make me stronger—rather, it helped me realize my strengths in new and different ways. My loss gave me new perspective and meaning, and through that, deeper spirituality and connections that have changed who I am as a person and physician. This took work and it is not linear. There are still days and weeks where I struggle, and when I do, I remind myself of the lessons I have learned. I try to be kind to myself and use compassionate language and thoughts when reflecting on my experiences. And most importantly, I still take life one moment at a time, in whatever increment of time I feel I can handle.

> Dr. Palamara McGrath's personal and professional mission has been to support the well-being of others through her work in physician well-being and coaching, and the nonprofit organization that she and her husband run in memory of their son—Colin's Joy Project. She has found exercise to be one of the most useful mechanisms for her grief and stressors in life and has run several marathons for Colin's Joy Project. When not working, you can find Dr. Palamara McGrath cheering their daughter Sloane on in one of her many sports, skiing with her family, or playing with their son Miles at one of the playgrounds built by Colin's Joy Project.

Mental Compartment Syndrome: It Is Time to Decompress

Imani E. McElroy

Zamoura and I were not able to share the childhood you would expect of siblings. He was raised by members of our biological family, whereas I became a ward of the state shortly after birth, before eventually being adopted. It would be over two decades before he and I would be reunited. Our first meeting was expectedly shy. We shared a quiet, easy-going nature that ultimately served as the foundation of our relationship. Soon after meeting, we began sending messages over social media and discovered a shared love of the creative arts, mainly sketching. Z, as we affectionately called him, would send videos of his daughters and pictures of his life events. I would share academic milestones and pictures of friends. Although raised separately, we were kindred spirit that bonded quickly and deeply.

Unfortunately, we would only share 7 years together. Z was murdered during my second year of surgical residency. In an instant, my world turned upside down. At the time, I did not recognize the depth of my grief—but losing Z would be the sentinel event that began an unraveling of my overworked mind. Up until his death, I had been able to walk the fine line of compartmentalization and decompression necessary to function in high-stress environments like surgical residency. It took me crying in the fetal position on a cold bathroom floor a year later to understand the importance of acknowledging trauma and stress before they become debilitating.

Early in my surgical training, I was taught to identify the warning signs of compartment syndrome: altered sensorium, loss of function, unrelenting pain. After an inciting trauma, a surgeon must act quickly to decompress the threatened area before irreversible complications occur. In some cases, we even perform prophylactic decompressive procedures, enabling the body to swell and heal more freely. Other times, the stressor is too great, resulting in massive cell and tissue death. Just as in the physical realm, emotional and psychological insults can trigger similar psychological cascades that can result in devastating consequences for the mind. Simple tasks become unmanageable, focus is fleeting, and emotional liability can force social isolation. In lay terms, we refer to this as a psychological breakdown.

Z's death was my significant stressor. As a junior trainee within a rigorous surgical residency, my desire to be perceived as "tough" coupled with avoidance of grief pushed me back to work just 1 week after his death. My program was able to find emergency coverage for me to fly home and likely could have given me another week, but the distractions work could provide and the guilt of knowing my colleagues were carrying an extra workload in my absence pulled me back into the hospital. So, I flew back into town and attempted to push away my grief and confusion by focusing on my work. In other words, I was compartmentalizing. But my mind was overpacked and there was nowhere for my grief to hide.

The more I tried to compress my emotions, the more my work suffered. For months, I stumbled through patient care in a fog, lagging on my previously diligent documentation. I became tentative and fearful in the operating room, and I grew increasingly frustrated with my inefficiency. I perceived these as weaknesses. Fear of failing exacerbated my underlying anxiety, and warning signs began to manifest. In the months after Z's death, I had panic attacks almost daily. Tearful outbursts, occasionally in public, came with increasing frequency. My impending collapse was predictable, and it occurred shortly before Z's birthday.

After rounds one morning, I became increasingly overwhelmed by routine questions from my intern. With each notification of a new message my heart raced, and my hands began to shake. As I tried to focus on answers, my mind failed me, and I could no longer recall dosing of routine meds or next steps in postoperative pathways. I rushed off to a private bathroom just outside our resident workroom. My grief became insurmountable, my legs finally gave under the pressure, and grief washed over me. I collapsed onto the bathroom floor and wept uncontrollably. Eventually, I reached a colleague who alerted the administrative chief residents to find someone to relieve me of my duties. The emotional trauma that I had tried so hard to suppress overloaded my system and transformed into physical inability.

Physicians—especially surgeons—experience secondary trauma as part of their job: intraoperative complications or death, severely injured patients, heroic measures to salvage life, starting a cancer operation only to find widely metastatic disease, comforting loved ones of lost patients. These insults increase the emotional pressure we feel, as we often place the burden of failure to save on ourselves as a personal defeat. We tuck away our grief to allow space for our patients and their families, only to move onto the next task on our ever-growing list of to-dos. We feel the pressure of our overworked health care system and the demands of meeting metrics without ever stopping to decompress. Like the muscle compartments in our body, swelling from trauma, we can only take so much pressure before something—our relationships, our tempers, our composure—becomes overwhelmed and fails.

The association between high levels of stress, depression, physician burnout, and suicide has been well documented in the literature—in one study, 1 in 16 surgeons reported suicidal ideation. However, most of these surgeons were unlikely to seek professional help due to fear of job-related repercussions. The impulse to suffer in silence among medical professionals, especially surgeons, has gone on for far too long and has resulted in too many untimely deaths. As we navigate the collective trauma of the COVID-19 pandemic on the healthcare system, the acknowledgement that we are collectively in need of better support has still not moved the needle sufficiently in terms of providing support for those who need it.

As we know from practice, the presence of symptoms in compartment syndrome signal that we are already behind in our treatment algorithm. Implementing a structured system to help mitigate the development of compartment syndrome is equally as important as promptly treating it once it develops. Peer support groups, on-call mental health professionals to assist with acute crises, regularly scheduled individual or group therapy sessions, and mandatory debriefing sessions after significant adverse outcomes are just the beginning in developing pressure-release valves for our trainees and staff.

The critical aspect of any support system will be normalizing the importance of decompression. Our "tough it out" mentality has left little room to develop healthy coping mechanisms or allow us the space to be human. We have failed ourselves as caregivers by upholding a system that is in direct contradiction with our teaching paradigms. Losing my brother has been life altering. Although I miss him dearly, in grieving him, I have gained perspective on what healing from significant trauma means. Luckily, I have been surrounded by friends and family willing to show up in uncomfortable moments consistently. I am grateful for their compassion because I otherwise might not be here to write this.

We owe it to our patients, families, and, most importantly, ourselves to prioritize our emotional well-being primarily before we show up to care for others. Through this process, I have learned not only the importance of early intervention but also that true strength is embracing the uncomfortable and messy parts of life. Allowing oneself to be vulnerable opens space to allow for healing and growth. Continuing to compartmentalize our experiences without relief only compounds trauma and eventually could lead to irreparable harm.

> Dr. McElroy is a chief resident in the Department of Surgery at Massachusetts General Hospital, who is dedicated to changing the narrative around mental health in the surgical workforce. She hopes that her work will change the overall tenor of how we talk about and make room for surgeons to express their own vulnerability in an otherwise tough work environment.

No Symptoms or Signs

Mark Allan Goldstein

It was one of those memorable autumn days: a cobalt blue cloudless sky, cool crispy air forecasting the coming of winter, and falling leaves whipped endlessly by wind. I found myself in a large dimmed room overflowing with young people. But it was eerily quiet. Some were silently sobbing, others were staring into space. My aging frail mother sat quietly, grasping tissues, eyes reddened, silently regarding me. As I sat down next to her, I noticed in the front of the room elevated on a platform a mahogany colored wooden casket. In it was lying my just turned 22-year-old nephew Jordan.

I first met Jordan at his brit milah—a Jewish ritual circumcision performed at the infant's age of 8 days. At that time, I had completed 4 weeks of medical school at Georgetown, and my family already considered me to be a doctor. Jordan's father, my brother-in-law, asked me to take the role of sandek that consists of holding the baby during the procedure, a position of high honor at a brit. And he said that I would also have other responsibilities for Jordan, but he did not elaborate. The mohel—a religious person trained to do the procedure—performed the circumcision. As is customary under Jewish tradition, once the brit is completed, an infant boy is named—generally after a deceased relative. In Jordan's case, it was my father's brother Julie. And then we enjoyed a celebratory meal.

Jordan was an exceptional child: humorous and popular, he did well academically, excelled in football and baseball, and was voted best all-around student in his high school class. And he also was a model citizen. He pledged a fraternity in college and was in a long-term relationship. After 2 years of college in Louisiana, Jordan transferred to Virginia Commonwealth University in Richmond.

Exactly 22 years to the day after I first met Jordan at his bris, he was driving to school from his home in northern Virginia, and he pulled his car over to the breakdown lane on Interstate 95. Jordan lifted the car's hood, and then he dashed into oncoming traffic. He left a suicide note, but no one now remembers the contents.

A few weeks after his funeral, I spoke at length with my sister. Were there any indications that Jordan was unhappy, depressed, feeling sad? Had his behavior or sleep changed recently? Were there any recent academic or social setbacks? My sister told me that there were no apparent symptoms or signs of suicidality.

But then for the first time, she divulged that Jordan was treated for depression in high school, completed a course of medication, and he was discharged from care.

While there were no symptoms or signs apparent to Jordan's family, perhaps he had been silently struggling. My sister and I never again spoke about Jordan. And I did not speak to friends and colleagues of his death until now.

It seems that if an individual dies by suicide, we repress their name, their accomplishments, their being: they cease to exist. There is silence. Family and friends never articulated "May his memory be a blessing." In contrast, if an adolescent dies from an accident or illness, their name and memories persist. Their life is honored.

The death of a child by suicide is devastating to the surviving family members. Within a year of Jordan's death, his grandmother—my mother—died from heart failure, his father passed away in 2 years with recurrent breast cancer that had been in remission for 20 years, and within 5 years his mother, my sister, succumbed to previously undiagnosed metastatic colon cancer. And a close family member was diagnosed with severe depression. I have always questioned if the guilt resulting from Jordan's suicide was linked to the death and depression of these relatives.

My fellowship training was in adolescent medicine where I learned that any youth could potentially be suicidal with minimal symptoms or signs of suicidality. One phone call from my sister or me might have prevented Jordan's death.

To help me deal with Jordan's death, I found it imperative to funnel my guilt into actions. With the background premise that any youth could potentially be suicidal without symptoms or signs, I regarded every youth in my medical practice as potentially suicidal, and if I were concerned, I would have no hesitation to provide care or refer to a higher level of care. And as much as possible, I would have family involved in the care of the patient. And I would make all efforts to educate my patients, their families, clinicians, and the public about adolescent suicidality in as many different ways as possible. Jordan's death needed to be transformed into saving lives.

One afternoon years later, a college student younger than Jordan, phoned me at my Mass General office and said that he needed to speak with me in person. He would not tell me his concern, but he did say he was safe and would come with his mother. Sensing the urgency in his voice, I agreed to see him that day before clinic started. After he arrived, I sat with him and he told me that his grades were plummeting, he felt isolated at school, and was very unhappy. And then he spoke about his plan to kill himself using a handgun in a wooded area near his home. With his mother, the three of us walked to the emergency room to be checked in, and he was admitted to a local psychiatric hospital where he underwent treatment for depression and suicidality. He subsequently did well in follow-up.

And, in years to come, there were many more adolescents and young adults in my practice that I found were suicidal and were referred for care with excellent outcomes. And no one under my care ever had a death by suicide.

Fifty-five years after the brit, I still do not understand the additional responsibilities my brother-in-law wanted me to assume for Jordan. Perhaps it was left open because no one knows where life will lead us. What I do know is that any adolescent is potentially suicidal, and regardless of how a child dies, their life should be honored and their memory should not be forgotten.

I have also seen that Jordan's death has saved lives. May his memory be a blessing.

> Dr. Goldstein is the author (with his wife Myrna) of *How Technology, Social Media, and Current Events Profoundly Affect Adolescents*, published by the Oxford University Press in 2024. In addition, he is the Editor-in-Chief of *Current Pediatrics Reports*. Dr. Goldstein is the proud grandfather of five wonderful grandchildren.

Learning to Live in an Alternate Universe

Maria Trent

Greg and I cooked together and had a beautiful Thanksgiving dinner with our family in November 2019. As usual, we went around the table and shared our gratitude. He shared how proud he was of our children and how much he loved me. Later that night, he also shared that he hadn't been feeling well, but I shouldn't worry because he had a doctor's appointment on Monday. He gave me a reassuring look; I patted him on the chest and then peacefully went to sleep.

As an early riser, I got up to busy myself and eventually asked my son to wake his dad so that he could set up the wheelchair ramp while I went to the nursing home 5 minutes away to meet my mother. She had been diagnosed with Alzheimer's dementia. We celebrated holidays twice—once on the actual day and the next business day—so that she could use public transportation for seniors with mobility issues. My 11-year-old son called me almost immediately after I left and said, "I can't wake up Daddy!" I did a U-turn on the road near my home and flew home. I attempted to resuscitate Greg by performing CPR while my son called EMS, and my 14-year-old daughter sat in his car, hoping he would wake up. When EMS arrived, they confirmed what I already knew despite my efforts to bring him back, begging him with each press on his chest—he was gone.

The unexpected, sudden, and somewhat traumatic loss of a spouse who was an incredible academic, musician, middle-aged athlete, writer, father, sports dad, life partner, and best friend whom you are actively loving is a tough pill to swallow in middle age. It just sucked the fun out of everything. I missed laughing about crazy things that happened during the day, attending events for our children, and having someone to zip my dress or get advice from. I mostly missed being hugged and hugging him back. Our family felt dramatically smaller, but we endured the subsequent Christmas holiday by escaping home and with support from family and friends.

Initially, I also worried about returning from bereavement to in-person clinical medicine, feeling like a bit of a failure, having not prevented Greg's death. I remember meeting my section chief for coffee and sitting there tearfully in the cafe, still not quite put back together, a week before my return. While he was reassuring as always, I still questioned whether my "sick versus not sick" meter was broken.

On my first day back, I saw multiple patients struggling with loss and grief among those on my schedule. Their stories were full of violent trauma, and their recoveries were stifled by a lack of resources, support, and their engagement in unhealthy coping strategies like substance use. I walked them through their emotions and behaviors using motivational interviewing to conjure ideas for improved coping in a way that brought their loved one to the center of their plan as inspiration rather than hurt. I leveraged the "ball in the box" analogy that had been so helpful for me so that they knew I understood their pain. It was the last day of rotation for the resident working with me, so she sent me a note telling me how powerful of an experience it had been to see patients with me that day and that I affirmed her future to be the kind of doctor who went beneath the surface to help patients. In many ways, being seen this way by her was transformative for me as a physician because someone could still see that I had value to patients and families. I was back! I also had new tools and a perspective that enabled me to connect with patients differently.

Just as we seemed to get into a rhythm, the COVID-19 pandemic completely sent us into an alternate universe at home, work, and the community. Raising two grieving teens now isolated from their robust school, music, and sports clubs was a challenge, as activity was a source of healing for them. As a health professional and "essential employee," the fear of getting sick and dying from a work exposure was a lingering daily gut check as we moved forward with caution. We were extra careful until more news about the mechanism of infection spread and protections that could be used to keep one safe. I engaged in telemedicine for only 3 months as a first strategy for survival but ultimately returned to in-person clinical medicine with my mask. My children eventually went to school and played sports in masks until we were all vaccinated, and the infection rates dwindled.

It has now been almost 4 years since Greg's death. We've survived the pandemic, and I've accomplished and grown so much personally and professionally during this time. Even so, I still mark the years by the day after Thanksgiving and reflect each year to continue to move forward with purpose. In my last reflection, I shared the following with friends:

> *True love does not fade, but since it's porous, grief periodically seeps through, reminding us of what we've lost when the rest of the world has turned the page.*
> *Resilience is exhausting, even for those who are strong.*
> *Animals are intuitive and a great comfort. Our pup forces me to exercise and always seems to know whose day was the hardest among the three of us.*
> *Scaffolding adolescents on the cusp of autonomy is necessary but scary. I am still learning how to walk through my fear to give them the grace they need to keep growing.*
> *My two 'firewalkers' are still standing, becoming forged like steel to become people with purpose.*
> *My Greg is present in them in ways that catch me in the moment.*
> *Life is short and unfair but also amazing and full of surprises when living with an open mind and heart.*
> *Work accomplishments are nice, but they no longer feed my soul. I must stay alert to experience the amazing moments and joyful surprises.*
> *The people who always loved us are planted and unwavering with the tide.*
> *When I'm done, I'm done—and it's ok.*
> *Thanksgiving is a better day, thanks to time and some wonderful people in our lives.*

Missing Greg, however, remains inescapable.
—Maria Trent, M.D., M.P.H.

In Loving Memory of Dr. Gregory Hampton, Ph.D., M.A.

> Dr. Trent is a pediatrician and specialist in adolescent and young adult medicine. Her work has focused on reducing sexual and reproductive health disparities among adolescents and young adults, as well as mentoring the next generation of adolescent health scientists. Through her clinical service, scientific endeavors, and organizational leadership, she has become an important advocate for adolescent and young adult health in the United States. Dr. Trent is the proud mother of two wonderfully resilient and talented young people who inspire her daily.

Superiority of the Grieving Syndrome (SGS)

Clara Baselga-Garriga

The names used in this story have been changed to protect their privacy.
My symptoms were gradual. A wave of irritation when Eliza complained about long work hours and burnout. An attempt to suppress an eye roll when Becca professed how torn she felt about whether to confront Julia about not inviting her to a dinner party "everyone" had gone to. A focused effort to stifle a yawn when Emily complained, again, about her boyfriend. I sat there, nodding my head, mumbling "I'm sorry" at socially acceptable intervals. I kept thinking: Don't they have real problems? These situations were reversible. The solutions weren't too complicated either: quit your job. Tell your friend you're annoyed—or don't (you can't attend a party that's already happened). And, for everyone's sake, dump the guy.

It's not like I lacked insight. I recognized I was being unfair. I was the type of person who requested the play-by-play of every single one of my friends' dates, knew their supervisors' worst traits, and where their siblings had applied for college early action. I was also no stranger to the anxieties associated with feeling drained by work and socially excluded which, given my flair for drama, felt like betrayal. My rational brain knew my friends had every right to air their grievances, but I couldn't stand it when they did.

Susan, my best friend's mother, *mhmm*-ed over the phone. Yes, there was no doubt about it. I had a bad case of SGS, or Superiority of the Grieving Syndrome. She had experienced this—and coined the term—herself back when her mom died. SGS, Susan explained, is triggered by losing a loved one and having to grapple with the irreversibility of death. In SGS, suffering acts like a moral cytokine, causing patients to develop a sense of superiority and irrational conviction that other's dilemmas are not in fact as complex or challenging as one's own because they are not dealing with death.

I lost my father in March 2021, 3 months after he was diagnosed with Creutzfeldt–Jakob disease, a one-in-a-million neurodegenerative, fatal illness. I remember the days around his death the way that I remember standardized tests—short intense moments of clarity and anxiety in a background of feverish blurriness. People came and went into the house to remind me to wake up, eat, and shower, like exam proctors marking the end of each exam section and the beginning of the next one.

I wore his dark grey quarter zip, the one he bought when we first moved to the United States, for days but couldn't bear to go near his copy of Watson's *The Double Helix*. I sustained myself on stale chips from half-emptied bags and diet Cokes. I feared our family would crumble after having lost a crucial link, but I didn't have the energy to engage in conversation with my brothers or mother. And then, there was this uncalled-for fury toward my friends. I was the one who had insisted they share their day-to-day with me for the sake of having some "normalcy," yet I despised it when they did.

Susan was right. I had packaged the messiness of grief—the haunting memories of his deterioration, the reality that he'd never see me in my white coat, or white dress—into simpler emotions: anger, hurt, and jealousy, all of it disguised in a sense of superiority. My subconscious had picked my fully parented, happy, and relentlessly supportive friends as the target of some of those feelings. SGS didn't explain all of my grief symptoms, but it did give me an anchor to begin to grasp some of the things I was experiencing. Twenty-four years of people-watching promised me grief in the form of wet tears and quiet longing. I experienced grief as disordered eating, panicked thoughts of my father's illness contaminating my memories of him, and the conviction that my pain was unequivocally worse than anyone else's.

I started medical school grieving and determined to learn all the things about grief that my body felt but could not make sense of. Physicians, too, seemed to have a hard time with this universal experience. In the 1950s, Sigmund Freud took a stab at it by putting grief into buckets: mourning was healthy; melancholy was maladaptive. In the 1970s, Elisabeth Kübler-Ross put grief into stages: denial, anger, bargaining, depression, and acceptance. In the 1990s, Holly Prigerson put grief into a scale: the Inventory of Complicated Grief. In 2019, the DSM-5 put Prolonged Grief Disorder (PGD) into its manual. It took over 60 years of putting grief into boxes of all sorts and sizes to come up with a diagnosis for an experience that has been around for as long as humans have felt loss.

To get the diagnosis of PGD, patients have to endorse, for at least 6 months, three of the following eight symptoms: disruption of identity, disbelief about the death, avoidance of reminders that the person is dead, intense emotional pain related to the death, difficulty with reintegration into life of the death, numbness, feeling that life is meaningless as a result of the death, and intense loneliness as a result of the death.

I counted how many of these symptoms I'd *endorsed* since my father died. To my relief, envy of those who hadn't lost loved ones wasn't included as one of the criteria. I was running out of fingers.

There was controversy around including PGD in the DSM-5. People were worried about the implications of pathologizing grief. They shared, in public forums, that grieving for 6 months wasn't abnormal, and that making prolonged grief a mental disorder may lead to stigma. I felt I somehow knew these people, and I bet they, too, had lost loved ones. I wondered whether their "inventory of grief" was also more like a dark abstract painting than a list. The DSM responded to this feedback by modifying the PGD criteria to require 12 months of intense yearning and preoccupation after a loved one's passing, plus 3 out of the 8 aforementioned symptoms. Even with the extension, grieving "appropriately" felt like an impossible task.

In our "Interview and Communication Skills" course during our first year of medical school, we were taught how to respond to challenging situations, including those pertaining to loss, by saying: "That must have been hard for you." The more you said it, the more brownie points you got on standardized patient interviews. The sentence always bothered me, but I couldn't vocalize why.

The wards brought some clarity. There, I witnessed grief as a third party in all of its shades—as all-encompassing anger, as demanding of MRI and CT scans, as desire to get the discharge documents prepared immediately, as deafening silence, as agreement to meet with the social worker, as resigned acceptance. I then realized that others couldn't possibly know whether one's grief was difficult or not, how it was difficult, why it was difficult, or for how long it may be difficult. When it came to grief, there was no such thing as the term "must."

Before I experienced grief, I had such a clear understanding of it. Grief was this concoction of emotions that happened over time when someone died. Grief's length and intensity was directly correlated with the proximity of the person who died. Grief was worse if the causational death was particularly tragic, surprising, dragged on over a long time, or if the relationship between the deceased and the grieving was complicated. Grief came in the same stages as *Teen Vogue*'s advice pieces on how to get over heartbreak. Before I experienced grief, I felt grief "must be hard" for those who experienced it.

Since I have grieved, I have lost my understanding of it. Today, all I know about grief is that you can never fully understand another person's grief, its manifestations, or its palliations. You may have SGS or PGD, or neither or both. You may find comfort in these labels or find them stigmatizing. Grief, people say, is universal. In medicine, it is an occurrence that physicians and patients alike are exposed to, sometimes perceived as an opportunity to foster patient–physician relationships. The problem is that, even though the concept of grief may be universal, *one's grief* is uniquely individual. Mine is still evolving every day. My SGS is somewhat in remission these days, but the thoughts of Nougat ice cream—his favorite—still makes me nauseated. As a future physician and caregiver, I am learning that there may be limitations to what I can say or do to help a grieving patient. I am learning all I may be able to offer is an "I'm sorry," an "I'm here," and a promise that I'll listen.

> Ms. Baselga-Garriga is a third-year medical student at Harvard Medical School, who obtained her Master of Fine Arts in Creative Nonfiction from Columbia University School of the Arts in 2021. She believes that stories have the power to foster understanding, increase access, and galvanize change in medicine. Her work has been featured in *El País*, *Intima*, and *In Vivo*, among others.

I Learned the Most from My Father's Death Following Surgery

Gleeson Rebello

I didn't stop running—from the day I started orthopedic residency until the day I finished it.

In a pre-cell phone and pre-electronic medical record era, I sprinted. I clocked in hundreds of thousands of unrecorded steps carrying information—for fellow clinicians, for patients, for their loved ones. The worst was bearing bad news—sometimes I felt I could barely catch my breath, even for those times, but I always managed to. I thought I was done with the marathon when I finished residency. Yet, once again, I found myself on the run, zipping from a well-known Mumbai hospital to a nearby hotel room. Once again, I was bearing bad news. But this time, the bad news wasn't for the family of one of my patients.

It was for my surgeon mother.

As I ran, pushing through the dense crowd, my senses stayed numb to the incessant cacophony of the traffic and its boundless supply of inescapable exhaust fumes. Mumbai, a bedazzling beehive of unabating human activity, suddenly seemed to have gone dark and come to a standstill.

But just for me.

Mom looked up as I entered the room. She appeared to be praying silently with the beads of the holy rosary trembling in her otherwise rock-steady hands. "Does the hospital need more cash?" she asked, nodding toward an open briefcase on the bed stacked with high denomination rupee notes. Like most Indians in the 1990s, we had to pay an advance in cash for treatment in big-city private hospitals and replenish the account when the deposit ran out.

She thought I had come to collect more money. I had come to give her the bad news.

The news that I carried with me followed my sudden exit from my 60-year-old dad's ICU bedside. He had undergone a cardiac bypass the previous day in the Mumbai hospital and was feeling uneasy. Uneasy enough that the Catholic in him asked for a priest to administer the last rites. I reassured him that he would be fine; nevertheless, I found a church nearby and a priest who was kind enough to drop everything and walk back to the hospital with me. I laughed through my nervousness as I said to the priest, "My dad is a very anxious man … so much for the steely confidence of a surgeon undergoing surgery!" Father Barbosa nodded with understanding, "He will feel better after I pray with him." We all prayed together by his bedside, and at the end, the priest anointed my dad's forehead with holy oil.

Dad and I were big fans of "famous last words" trivia and overdone Bollywood movies where characters that knew they were going to die both bled and gasped out a whole last will and testament. Possibly our final exchange would have been longer and more poignant had we known what was to follow. Maybe, I would have never left his side. All I managed was a brusque, "Dad, I am going to walk Father Barbosa to the hospital entrance and will be back soon." He nodded, "I will be waiting," he said.

When I returned to my dad's hospital room, however, I walked into the all-too-familiar hell that breaks loose when a soul in hospital threatens to leave this world where a beeping storm of monitors triggers circumferential waves of quick-thinking human activity around a patient's bed. One of the humans by my dad's bedside was a young ICU resident who, 2 hours prior, had taken me aside and said, "We have run all the tests. Everything seems fine. I think your dad is a little anxious." Now, it was she who looked more than a little anxious.

The surgeon in me wanted to stay, but the son in me took over, and I began my lonely run back to the hotel.

I burst into the hotel room to break the news to Mom. Deep down inside, I knew that Dad had passed away, but my words came out clothed in a white coat, "Mom, Dad's condition suddenly got critical." Her eyes widened in shock. "Oh my God," she gasped. I pushed on, "I hope to God he makes it." My stricken face gave my words away.

As a physician herself, she did not need a bad news translator. "What's the use of all this?" she choked as she despairingly shoved the open briefcase filled with money from the bed onto the ground, where the notes ended up forming a bizarre-looking rug. Her hands continued to clutch the holy rosary. I didn't say anything more and just held her close.

Surgeons don't cry, they say. We both did—not just because another surgeon died but because a husband and father did.

We were both oblivious to the rupee notes scattered all over the ground. My Mom did not let go of the rosary beads. And we did not let go of each other. That moment drove home for me that when matters of sickness and health reach a point of reckoning, science and wealth may not necessarily be the highest power that the afflicted turn to, including the people of science who also possess wealth. Maybe it is because science does not always get it right, and money cannot cure every wrong.

As we stood desperately holding each other, I knew what was going on in my mind was possibly going on in hers, and we will never stop playing it in a loop, forever—the events and the decisions that led to our being here.

It all began when my otherwise asymptomatic dad consulted a doctor for throat burn after eating spicy food. This seemingly innocuous decision put him on a cascading investigative path in which an electrocardiogram led to a stress test led to an angiogram, a test that outlines the pipes that supply blood to the heart. This test demonstrated near-total blockage of the blood vessels that supplied his heart. Cardiac bypass surgery was recommended, but my dad wanted to have a balloon angioplasty, a procedure that can be performed by slipping a small tube through a hole poked in his thigh, as he did not want his "chest split open" by the surgery. The irony was not lost to me that surgeons are as afraid of surgery as everyone else—perhaps even more so.

Meanwhile, my non-medical uncle was symptomatic with constant chest pain. His angiogram was strikingly similar to my father's, and he, too, was recommended a cardiac bypass. Instead, he attended a weeklong religious retreat. During a healing session, the priest raised his arms heavenwards and thunderingly announced to the ten-thousand strong congregation, "In the name of God, ten people with heart disease among you have been cured of your ailment!" My uncle decided he was one of the chosen ten. Twenty-five years later, he is still alive. Maybe one does not always have to make the cut to make the cure as we surgeons like to think.

Given my father's angiography findings, his cardiologist did not recommend balloon angioplasty, as it had the potential to precipitate a block in the blood supply to the heart, lead to a heart attack, and necessitate an emergency bypass. But one of the country's foremost angioplasty experts who prided himself on his ability to do "cases that no one else has the ability to do" decided to give my father—"the patient"—what he wanted. My father ended up getting that forewarned complication and needing an emergency bypass. The interventional cardiologist possessed a hammer, and my dad asked to be the nail. The hammer-nail cliché had dealt yet another blow, this time too close to home. And in a crazy way, our family full of surgeons unwittingly aided the system in carving out our very own Swiss-cheese model of accident causation, creating perfectly aligned craters of calamity through which, holding hands, we executed a free fall.

At every point, Mom and I went with the flow, blindly trusting what the system had to offer and the decisions being made and going along with what my dad wanted. Adding to the calculus, elementally, we were from a "small town" and had come to the "big city" for treatment. To frame our medical journey using American geography, we lived in idyllic northern Maine and had traveled to a medical mecca comparable to Boston or New York City for my dad's treatment, where he ended up being treated by doctors of great renown who counted heads of state and Bollywood stars among their patients. Perhaps the humanity of big-name hospitals and rock-star physicians can be layered with an intimidating gloss that can make the awe-struck patient reluctant to subject that gloss to the nicks of questioning—even if the patient is a surgeon himself.

I have often wondered how the cardiac surgeon mentally processed my dad's death. I can imagine the well-meaning, yet clumsy, attempts of his colleagues to console him, akin to what well-meaning friends do to console at times of personal grief. "You did everything you could." "If you operate enough, you are going to have complications." "It could have happened to any of us."

All surgeons know the pain of having hurt someone we are trying to heal. We talk about our complications with our colleagues like we would talk with a close friend about a breakup or a death in the family. We are always deeply torn inside and wondering what we could have done differently and better. I think of that resident sometimes—the one who called him "anxious" 2 hours before he died. Just as I learned something, I hope she did, too. Wisdom that she will pass on to her trainees and that her patients will benefit from.

As a surgeon trainee in my mid-20s in an insanely busy environment with constraints and relatively limited supervision that accompanied orthopedic residency in my government-run university hospital in India circa 1990s, I would consider younger me as brash, overconfident, and at times even gung-ho. Moreover, it was considered a weakness to ask for assistance from one's senior colleague and displaying any type of vulnerability was utterly off the table. Surgeons and even trainee surgeons just didn't do that!

This attitude resulted in a public perception that we surgeons think we are God, and at times we are ridiculed for it. Truth be told that when faced with a complication, it is the one time we wish that we were a deity gifted with the power to change the course of events.

To our family of mortal surgeons, a well-intentioned system filled with kind and knowledgeable professionals delivered a death by a thousand cuts. We learned that when we are cut, we bleed just like everyone else.

I learned that a knife that carves you or your kin's body could also reshape your thinking and change your process of decision-making. It certainly did mine and made me more thoughtful whenever the opportunity arose to use a knife. Even though the timing of this tragedy could not have been worse for my family, it was, in a perverse way, beneficial for my future patients. Having recently completed my orthopedic residency, I now sat atop the decision-making tree that controlled life and limb, where a labor of planning, precision, and love could still yield the bitter fruit of failure. My indications to perform surgery especially in an elective situation became progressively tighter and the scales that balanced risk and reward worked ceaselessly in my hands. It fetched mixed reactions from my peers. There were those that respected and referred to my approach as thoughtful. And there were others who considered it in an extreme sense, diffident and un-surgeon like.

In an instant, this story of life, love, and loss produced a paradigm shift within me. It took many years for me to put my fingers to a keyboard and blink away my tears and share this story as I had yet to understand that it was OK to be both vulnerable and a surgeon. And it was going to take time to process this new direction in my personal evolution. I felt like a pre-historic life form where the asteroid had hit the ground beneath my feet and somehow, I had survived. My knees and legs were a little wobbly, yet my heart stayed beating, and my brain, which should have gotten numb, was getting to a place of even greater clarity than ever before. While I stayed on life's great hunt that was needed to ensure my continued existence as a human being and a surgeon.

From a narcissistic, egoistical, and immature surgeon who thought that only making the cut could result in the cure, my father's death helped me understand that there was a consequence that sprung from every action of mine. And that it could result in a person or even an entire family remembering me and not very fondly as they went through every activity of daily living in their otherwise seemingly mundane lives.

Some of us surgeons believe in the afterlife. I do. I hope my dad is listening in when I say, "Dad, I learned a lot in medical school and residency. I learned even more about what it means to be a doctor when you were alive, but sadly I learned the most from your death. Wherever you are, I want you to know that by constantly endeavoring to do the right thing by the patient, I am doing the right thing by you."

I know I will not always get it right, but it will never stop me from trying.

Dr. Rebello is a pediatric orthopedic surgeon, a children's book author, and a songwriter for the band The Fever Breakers. He believes that everyone's individual story collectively results in the world going round. A version of this essay by Dr. Rebello appeared on KevinMD.com.

Acknowledgements

Mark Allan Goldstein and Kathy May Tran

More than a year ago, we began to develop the idea for a book of essays written by doctors, residents, and medical students, which describes how they approached a challenge and how that process made them better doctors. From concept to creation, this work has brought us great joy. We owe a great deal of gratitude to those who helped us with this endeavor. These acknowledgements are not exhaustive.

Suzanne Koven, the Writer-in-Residence at Massachusetts General Hospital (MGH), supported this project from its beginning, and we are deeply grateful for her enthusiasm and endorsement. We thank Susan Hata at MGH and Randi Hutter Epstein at Yale, who suggested possible contributors. We are grateful to Max Schermer, a senior at Harvard College, for advice on illustrations. Thanks also to Fatima Cody Stanford and Kerri Palamara McGrath at MGH for supporting this project from its inception.

We are indebted to Richard Lansing, clinical medicine editorial director at Springer Nature, who has been most enthusiastic about this project and has provided wise guidance for its development. Our thanks to Julia Andrews, clinical medicine editor at Springer, who has given input and counsel about the format of this book. Henry Rodgers, project coordinator at Springer, has made certain that the production process flowed smoothly. And we have special thanks to Sharath Rangaraj, our production editor at Springer Nature, with whom we have had almost daily discussions about this book. Sharath demonstrated enormous patience with us.

Myrna Chandler Goldstein and Luther Warren, independent scholars and writers, have critiqued and provided input for many of the essays. For that advice and for their encouragement, we are very grateful.

We want to express appreciation to our families, friends, mentors, and colleagues who have remained steadfast in support of this work.

We wish to thank the contributors. They have shown great courage in writing about sensitive and personal topics such as prejudice, addiction, illness, adversity, caring for the dying, and agony from tragedy. As we worked closely with each contributor, we were inspired. Their stories of vulnerability, struggle, emotion, celebration, and success have taught us by example.

Finally, we want to thank you—the readers—who are interested in doctoring and who may be doctors or doctors-to-be yourselves. This community is the reason why this collection was conceived and brought to fruition. Thank you for reading our stories and thank you for helping us to become better physicians.

Index

A
Absolute neutrophil count (ANC), 10
Addiction, 76–79, 89
Age-appropriate vaccines, 35
Aggressive, 11
Alzheimer's dementia, 118
Anger, 4, 7
Angioplasty, 125
Antibiotics, 61
Anxiety, 4, 25, 26, 35, 39
Art of Listening, 45–50
Artificial intelligence, 54
Authenticity, 113
Autoimmune connective tissue disease, 72
Autonomy, 36

B
Ball in box analogy, 119
Barriers, 47
Behavioral health problems, 98
Bilingual capacity, 32
Boston pediatric residency program, 81
Breast cancer screening, 96
Buprenorphine, 78
Burnout, 92

C
Cancer, 32, 68, 106
Cardiac bypass surgery, 124
Cardiothoracic surgery, 51
Cardiovascular disease, 32
Career development, 28, 29, 32, 37, 38, 58
Career in medicine, 6
Caregivers, 61, 66
Caretakers, 66
Chemotherapy, 54

Child abuse, 19
Chronic disease, 81
Clinical reasoning, 44
Clinical trials, 33
Coalition, 35
Communication, 19, 27, 31, 33, 87
Communication skills, 87
Communication skills training, 72
Compartmentalization by physicians, 114
Compassion, 35
Compassion in doctor patient
    relationship, 65
Compassionate hemodialysis, 96
Competitive residency program, 37
Conflict, 38
Congenital anomaly, 69
Conscience, 32
Contingency management, 78
Contradictory emotions, 69
COVID epidemic, 85
Covid-19, alpha, 58
COVID-19 pandemic, 7, 14, 20, 21, 31–33,
    43, 45, 58, 98, 112, 115, 119
Covid-19 test, 58
COVID vaccine, 20
Cranial nerves, 96
Creutzfeldt-Jakob disease, 120
Criminal justice system, 77, 79
Critical illnesses, 54
Critically ill neonate, 69
Cultural competence, 34
Cultural differences, 47

D
Deferred Action for Childhood Arrivals
    (DACA), 96
Deficiencies, errors, and frustrations (DEF), 22

Dementia, 60
Demyelinating disease, 80
Depression, 39, 66, 78, 115, 116
Diabetes, 32, 78
Diagnostic criteria, 70
Diagnostic tests, 48
Doctor-adolescent-family partnership, 35
Doctor-patient relationship, 49, 50, 64, 65
Down syndrome, 55
Drug use, 39

E
Educational responsibilities, 30
Effectiveness of clinical care, 33
Electronic Medical Record (EMR) documentation, 7
Electronic Medical Record System, 38
Emergency medicine, 6
Emotional dysregulation, 35
Empathic family, 39
Empathy, 8, 35, 46
Employment-at-will, 23
End-of-life care, 60
Essential employee, 119
Exhaustion during residency, 8

F
Financial resources, 79
Freedom of speech, 24
Frustration of musician turned physician, 100–103

G
Gender inequalities, 19
Grief, 67, 122
    after loss, 110–113
    from patient care, 4–6
    stages, 121
    symptoms, 121

H
Health care, 22, 23, 33
Healthcare issues, 24
Health care providers, 88
Health care system, 7, 38, 47, 97
Health care workers, 66
Health insurance, 96
Health professional, 119
Health-services research, 7
Health system, 38

Hope, 124–126
Hyperkalemia, 96
Hypertension, 78
Hypoallergic sunscreens, 29

I
Ibuprofen, 71
Immigration, 97
Indigenous health advocacy partnerships, 13
Infection, 94
Infectious diseases, 25
In-person clinical medicine, 118

J
Job loss, 40
Joy Machine, 73–75

L
Laceration, 94
Language barriers, 97
Leadership responsibilities, 28
Leadership's decision, 23
Learning process, 3
Life-long learning, 82
Life-threatening illness, 83
Loss of a loved one, 115, 121
Love, 113, 119, 126
Lupus, 70

M
Mandatory assimilation program, 12
Marriage during residency, 13–16
Massachusetts Physician Health Service, 78
Massive sense of loss, 38
Mastery, 67
Medical advice, 51
Medical education research, 8
Medical intensive care unit (MICU), 43
Medical practice, 78
Medical professionals, 77
Medical school education, 4, 11–13
Medical training, 3, 5, 67
Mediocrity, 22
Melanoma, 68
Memory disorders, 43
Mental compartment syndrome, 113–116
Mental health, 49
Mental health team, 35

Mental illness, 48
Mentorship, 3, 7
Metabolic problems, 46
Microaggressions, 21
Monitored Academic Status, 11
Moods, 39
Moral injury, 32–34
Morbidity, 64
Mother's vaccination, 19
Multilingual registry of clinicians, 31
Multiple sclerosis, 81, 82
Music theory, 103

N
Narrative medicine, 11, 27, 72
Neurological diseases, 103
Neutrophil, 10
Nonadherence, 54

O
Oncology, 2, 9
Opioids, 106
Overcoming overwhelm, 97–100
Oxycontin, 76
Oxygen saturation, 56

P
Painkillers, 76
Palliative care, 9
    community, 6
    physician, 10–11
Palliative chemotherapy, 2
Pathophysiology, 36
Patient care, 46, 47, 55, 57
Patient-caregiver relationships, 46
Patient safety, 22
Peer support groups, 115
Personal growth, 92–107
Personal relationships, 15
Physician advocacy, 24
Physician burnout, 115
Physician Health Service (PHS), 78, 79
Pneumonitis, 55
Posttraumatic growth-of surviving, 113
Primary care, 44, 45
    physician, 97
    provider, 22
Professional development, 30
Professional identities, 37
Professionalism concerns, 11
Professionalism in medicine, 8–11

Professionalism training program, 12
Prolonged Grief Disorder (PGD), 121
Promotions and review board (PRB), 11
Prophylactic decompressive procedures, 114
Pursued music therapy, 102

R
Racial-ethnic backgrounds, 81
Refrigerator mothers, 20
Refuge, 44, 45
Rehabilitation program, 39
Reputation, 30
Residency training, 10, 15

S
SARS-CoV-2, 58
Schizophrenogenic mothers, 20
Secondary trauma, 115
Self-care, 30
Self-compassion, 66
Self-preservation, 107
Self-promotion, 30
Serious illness, 69
Social health, 54
Socioeconomic needs, 54
Spanish Language Care Group (SLCG), 32, 33
State-of-the-art procedure, 86, 87
Stethoscope, 81
Storytellers, 3
Streptococcal pharyngitis, 80
Stress, 4, 112, 115
Suboxone, 78, 79
Substance abuse, 67
Substance use disorder, 66
Success, 29, 30
Suicidality, 116, 117
Suicide, 117
Suicide of relative, 117
Superiority of the Grieving Syndrome (SGS), 120
Systematic disenfranchisement, 29
Systems-level change, 7

T
Technical training, 81
Telemedicine, 119
"Tell Me More" project, 54–57
Tender care, 45
Tenderness, 45
Tenuous optimism, 72

Tragedy, 126
Transition phase, 35
Trauma, 37
Trauma-informed care, 95
Turbulent adolescence, 34
Turner syndrome, 46
Two-way communication, 88

U
Uncompassionate caregivers, 35
Unconscious biases, 19
Undocumented medicine, 95–97
Unethical conduct, 19
Unintentional process, 77
Unrelenting standards, 99
Uremic symptoms, 96

V
Vaccination, 19, 21
    risks and benefits of, 20
Vaccine, 36
Vaccine advocacy, 21
Ventricular assist device (VAD), 51, 52
Vertigo, 64
Vicodin, 76
Visual thinking strategies, 72
Vulnerability, 125

W
With limited-English proficiency (LEP), 31
Work-life balance, 27–30
World Economic Forum, 20
Writing by physicians, 76

MIX
Papier aus verantwortungsvollen Quellen
Paper from responsible sources
FSC® C105338

If you have any concerns about our products,
you can contact us on
ProductSafety@springernature.com

In case Publisher is established outside the EU,
the EU authorized representative is:
**Springer Nature Customer Service Center GmbH
Europaplatz 3, 69115 Heidelberg, Germany**

Printed by Libri Plureos GmbH
in Hamburg, Germany